Monographs on Endocrinology

Volume 13

H. F. DeLuca

Vitamin D
Metabolism and Function

With 14 Figures

Springer-Verlag
Berlin Heidelberg New York 1979

Dr. Hector F. DeLuca

Department of Biochemistry,
College of Agricultural and Life Sciences,
University of Wisconsin – Madison,
Madison, Wisconsin 53706 – USA

ISBN-13: 978-3-642-81308-5 e-ISBN-13: 978-3-642-81306-1
DOI: 10.1007/ 978-3-642-81306-1

Library of Congress Cataloging in Publication Data.
DeLuca, Hector F. 1930–
Vitamin D. (Monographs on endocrinology; v. 13)
Bibliography: p. Includes Index. 1. Vitamin D. 2. Vitamin D metabolism. I. Title.
QP772.V53D44 612'.399 79-677

Typesetting: R. Leipe, Hagenbach

2125/3020 – 543210

Acknowledgments

Some of the original investigations reported in this chapter were supported by a program-project grant No. AM-14881 from the National Institutes of Health, and the Harry Steenbock Research Fund of the Wisconsin Alumni Research Foundation.

Contents

A. **Introduction** 1

B. **Historical Aspects** 3

C. **The D Vitamins and Their Precursors** 8

D. **Metabolism of Vitamin D** 11

- I. Absorption of Vitamin D_3 11
- II. Production of Vitamin D in the Skin 11
- III. Storage of Vitamin D 13
- IV. Role of the Liver in Production of 25-Hydroxyvitamin D_3 . . 13
- V. Metabolism of 25-Hydroxyvitamin D_3 to 24,25-Dihydroxyvitamin D_3 17
- VI. Production of 1,24,25-Trihydroxyvitamin D_3 19
- VII. Other Metabolites of Vitamin D_3 20
- VIII. Metabolism of Vitamin D_2 and Dihydrotachysterols 21

E. **Regulation of Vitamin D Metabolism: The Kidney as an Endocrine Organ** 24

- I. Regulation of 25-Hydroxyvitamin D_3 Production 24
- II. Regulation of 1,25-Dihydroxyvitamin D_3 Production by Calcium and Parathyroid Hormone 25
- III. Regulation of 1,25-Dihydroxyvitamin D_3 Metabolism by Serum Phosphorus Concentration 28
- IV. Regulation of 25-Hydroxyvitamin D_3-24-Hydroxylase by 1,25- Dihydroxyvitamin D_3, Parathyroid Hormone, and Ambient Calcium Concentration 28
- V. Regulation of Vitamin D Metabolism by the Sex Hormones . 29
- VI. Mechanisms of Regulation of the Renal Hydroxylases . . . 30
- VII. Calcium Homeostatic Mechanisms Involving the Vitamin D Endocrine System 31

F. **Functions of Vitamin D** 35

- I. Intestine 35
  1. Calcium Transport 35
  2. Factors which Regulate Intestinal Calcium Transport by Regulating Vitamin D Conversion to 1,25-$(OH)_2D_3$ . . . 39

3. The Molecular Mechanism of Action of 1,25-$(OH)_2D_3$ in Intestinal Calcium Transport 41
4. Intestinal Phosphate Transport 47
5. Stimulation of Intestinal Calcium Transport by Phosphate Deprivation 47
II. Functions of Vitamin D in Bone 48
1. Mineralization 48
2. Bone Calcium Mobilization 49
3. Other Possible Roles of Vitamin D in Bone 50
III. Kidney 50
IV. The Function of Vitamin D in Muscle and Elsewhere 51

G. Analogs of 1,25-Dihydroxyvitamin D_3 and 25-Hydroxyvitamin D_3 . 53
I. Analogs of 25-Hydroxyvitamin D_3 53
II. 1α-Hydroxyvitamin D_3 and 1α-Hydroxyvitamin D_2 54
III. 3-Deoxy-1α-Hydroxyvitamin D_3 and 3-Deoxy-1,25-Dihydroxyvitamin D_3 55
IV. Other Analogs of Vitamin D 55

H. Use of Vitamin D Compounds in Medicine, Especially 1,25-Dihydroxyvitamin D_3 57

J. Summary and Conclusions 60

References 61

Subject Index 79

A. Introduction

Because diseases of the bone are often less acute and less lifethreatening than diseases of the circulatory system, gastrointestinal tract, kidney, liver, and the nervous system, they have received a disproportionately smaller amount of attention in the medical world. With the average increasing life span of man as a result of improvements in modern medicine, especially in the pediatric field, the seriousness of many metabolic bone diseases has indeed become more obvious. In addition, other improvements in medicine, such as hemodialysis for the preservation of renal failure patients, have permitted the development of other consequences of diseased kidneys, one of which is the appearance of renal osteodystrophy. Finally, the appearance of several genetic disorders in the area of metabolic bone disease has been underscored by the solution of other pediatric diseases of much more serious consequences. These emerging problems all suggest that much remains to be learned concerning the systemic control of bone, both as a structural organ and as a reservoir for the important elements of calcium and phosphorus so essential for the support of life in complex multicellular organisms of which man is the most important.

As will be demonstrated in the historical portion of this manuscript, the existence of the three most important humoral factors regulating bone metabolism and function are now known. One of these, termed vitamin D, has been known since 1920 as a chemical and scientific entity and perhaps longer as a medical factor, yet its role has only recently been defined in any satisfactory manner. The factor, which is termed antirachitic factor or vitamin D, can be considered a vitamin only in the sense that man has, during the course of the last 4,000–5,000 years, changed his life style so that he now does not receive adequate amounts of ultraviolet irradiation of solar origin. Because of scientific investigations during the past 50 years, we recognize that this resulted in a failure of production of the important humoral factor (vitamin D), which could be replaced by dietary consumption of such foods as fish-liver oils or irradiated plant materials. This factor, upon isolation and identification, was termed vitamin D, but it must be recognized that it truly is not a vitamin if man receives sufficient amounts of ultraviolet light so that it can be produced in sufficient quantities in the skin. During the past decade, with the introduction of modern biochemical techniques including chromatography, chemical synthesis of radioactive forms of the vitamin of high specific activity, and the use of mass spectrometry and nuclear magnetic resonance spectroscopy, we have learned that this substance is in fact a precursor of at least one hormone that functions in the regulation of calcium and phosphorus metabolism.

This monograph is an attempt to bring together the salient features of the vitamin D metabolic system as it is currently understood. Of great importance is the possibility that the hormonal form of vitamin D and its analogs can be used in the treatment of a variety of metabolic disorders induced either by the failure of a particular organ or by genetic means. It is also possible that one of the senescent processes involves a deterioration of the vitamin D endocrine system, which may give rise in part to the development of bone disease related to the aging process. Finally, it should be recognized that this monograph is in a sense a progress report of a study of the metabolism and function of vitamin D and its implications in medicine and that the findings reported here are likely, during the next decade, to be supplanted by more sophisticated information that will define more clearly the calcium and phosphorus homeostatic mechanisms, thereby giving the treatment of metabolic bone diseases a scientific base and rendering it more effective.

B. Historical Aspects

The importance of sunlight to the sturdiness of the skeletal structure was alluded to even in ancient times (HESS, 1929). The apparently softer skulls of Persians compared to those of Egyptians were discerned in the field of battle. It is possible that the Egyptians, who shaved their hair and wore scanty clothing, permitted ultraviolet light to be incident on their skin, whereas the Persians, who wore turbans and covered much of their bodies, prevented ultraviolet light from reaching their skin. Possibly, vitamin D was not produced in sufficient quantities, resulting in thinner bones. Whether or not this actually occurred is a matter of speculation. However, there are writings throughout recorded history of debilititating bone disease that might well have been related to inadequate irradiation by sunlight because of religious or cultural practices or because of the life style (HESS, 1929). Whatever the speculation, at least in modern recollection, the first true description of a bony disease considered to be rickets was by Glisson in 1650 or by Whistler in 1645 (HESS, 1929). The bony lesions of rickets were described in increasing detail over the next several centuries, but it was not until the 1900s when the disease rickets was given a scientific basis (MELLANBY, 1919a and b).

There is much controversy concerning the origin of the term rickets. In one school of thought, rickets is believed to arise from the term rucket, meaning to breathe with difficulty, probably because breathing was impaired because of improper rib development (HESS, 1929; NICOLAYSEN and EEG-LARSEN, 1953). Another school holds that the word rickets came from the Welch term "wrygates", which meant crooked goings or twisted legs (NICOLAYSEN and EEG-LARSEN, 1953). Other theories have appeared (HESS, 1929) but in any case it should be recognized that rickets is a disease that has been recognized for many centuries, and in fact some of the methods for curing the disease were alluded to long before scientific investigation. Thus cod liver oil was utilized to treat the disease, and fresh air and sunlight were also mentioned in old wives' tales (HESS, 1929). However, it was not until the turn of the century, when the concept of vitamins came into focus, that one could begin to understand the disease rickets and could recognize the existence of an antirachitic factor. Some of the basic work leading to the discovery of the vitamins must be attributed to LIEBIG (1841), to MAGENDIE (1816), and to HOPKINS (1906), who reasoned that, knowing the chemical composition of foodstuffs, it should be possible to support life with those purified chemicals. However, each of these investigators failed to support life with purified mixtures of carbohydrate, protein, fat, and minerals. FUNK introduced the concept of "vital amines", which would be necessary to support life and reproduction of animals (FUNK, 1911). EICHMANN found that polished white rice led to the appearance of beri-beri in populations of prisoners in the Dutch East Indies, and furthermore that this could be prevented by adding back the rice polishings (EICHMANN, 1897). Although he incorrectly concluded that this was the result of a toxic factor introduced by polishing of rice, his colleague, GRIJNS, later came to the correct conclusion and reasoned that a factor that prevented beri-beri must be present in rice hulls (GRIJNS, 1935). HOLST and FRÖLICH (1907) demonstrated that scurvy could be prevented or cured by the juice of fresh limes or other fresh vegetables and thus discovered vitamin C.

From a practical point of view, the group at the Wisconsin Agricultural Experiment Station found that fodders of equal composition but from either wheat, or oats had differential life-supporting properties in dairy cattle, corn being superior and wheat being the most inferior. They postulated the existence of micronutrients, heretofore unknown, that were necessary for life (HART et al., 1911). This led to the development of a small animal colony at that institution that led to Professor McCollum carrying out his classical experiments in which he demonstrated the existence in butterfat and cod liver oil of a factor that was essential to the growth and health of animals (MCCOLLUM and DAVIS, 1913). This factor he called fat-soluble vitamin A (MCCOLLUM et al., 1916). Similar work was carried out at the Connecticut Experiment Station with Professors OSBORNE and MENDEL, and almost simultaneously, the presence of water-soluble vital factors, which MCCOLLUM named water-soluble vitamin B, was discovered (MCCOLLUM et al., 1916; OSBORNE and MENDEL, 1917). Thus this series of investigations ushered in the concept of microorganic nutrients that were essential to growth and development of animals. It is in this setting that Sir Edward Mellanby began his work on the discovery of the antirachitic substance. Sir Edward Mellanby, undoubtedly inspired by the development of the vitamins and by MCCOLLUM's work, attempted to reproduce the, at that time, widespread disease by experimental or nutritional maneuvers. Parenthetically, it should be noted that the industrial revolution ushered in a high incidence of rickets in the population centers of Europe and North America, primarily because of the marginal sunlight in those areas due to the presence of large amounts of smoke and air pollution, which undoubtedly prevented ultraviolet light from reaching the skin of children, and furthermore due to spending more time indoors, which also prevented exposure to ultraviolet light (HESS, 1929). This led to the appearance of rickets in epidemic proportions in most of the northern temperate zone. In any case, SIR EDWARD MELLANBY was able to produce a disease in dogs that closely resembled rickets found in children (MELLANBY, 1919a; 1919b). He was able to prevent or cure that disease with cod liver oil, and because MCCOLLUM had found fat-soluble vitamin A in cod liver oil, Sir Edward Mellanby concluded that fat-soluble vitamin A prevents or cures the disease rickets. Although the latter conclusion may have been incorrect, the discovery of Sir Edward Mellanby that rickets could be produced experimentally and that dietary factors could prevent the disease placed the investigation of vitamin D on a truly scientific basis. MCCOLLUM, who had been concerned with fat-soluble vitamin A for some time, recognized that the properties of the antirachitic substance discovered by Sir Edward Mellanby must be different from those of the growth-promoting fat-soluble vitamin A. By bubbling oxygen through cod liver oil and heating it, he was able to destroy the vitamin A or growth-promoting activity while retaining the ability to prevent or cure rickets (MCCOLLUM et al., 1922). He therefore reasoned that this must be a new fat-soluble vitamin, which he then called vitamin D. In Vienna, however, another series of investigations was taking place at the clinical level. HULDSHINSKY (1919) and CHICK et al. (1923) independently demonstrated that exposure of rachitic children to sunlight or artificially induced ultraviolet light prevented or cured their disease. Therefore, in

1922–1923, the field was confused because both cod liver oil and sunlight prevented rickets. Insight into this problem was provided by the experiments of GOLDBLATT and SOAMES (1923), who showed that ultraviolet irradiation of rachitic rats resulted in a factor in the liver that could be extracted and could cure other rachitic rats. Thus ultraviolet light produced the antirachitic factor in rachitic animals. However, STEENBOCK provided the first established and sound basis of ultraviolet activation of provitamin Ds. In a classical series of investigations, he clearly showed that ultraviolet irraditation not only of animal skins but also of their food introduced into those substances antirachitic activity (STEENBOCK, 1924; STEENBOCK and BLACK, 1924). This work, which was confirmed by HESS and WEINSTOCK (1924), was then extended by both groups to demonstrate that the activatable factor is found in the nonsaponifiable or sterol fraction (STEENBOCK and BLACK, 1925; HESS et al., 1926). These discoveries laid the groundwork for the isolation and identification of the D vitamins and led to the elimination of rickets as a major medical problem in the western world. By irradiation of food initially, especially milk, one could introduce vitamin D in a harmless fashion and thus eliminate the problem of rickets. The isolation and identification of the D vitamins was the next important development in this area. WINDAUS and his colleagues were the first to isolate a crystalline substance that they termed vitamin D_1. In retrospect vitamin D_1 proved to be an artifactual addition product of vitamin D_2 and a contaminating sterol lumisterol (WINDAUS and LINSERT, 1928). This development undoubtedly slowed the activity of the WINDAUS group and permitted ASKEW and colleagues to first clearly identify the first antirachitic substance, isolated from solutions of the irradiated plant sterol ergosterol (ASKEW et al., 1931). This work was completed in 1932, providing the first identification of a vitamin D. At almost the same time WINDAUS and his colleagues provided identical evidence for the vitamin derived from ergosterol (WINDAUS et al., 1932). This vitamin, which is now known as ergocalciferol or vitamin D_2, was for many years the major synthetic form of vitamin D used for the prevention and cure of rickets in man. STEENBOCK and his colleagues, in a continuing investigation, noted that birds did not react well to solutions of irradiated ergosterol when compared to either cod liver oil or solutions of irradiated cholesterol (STEENBOCK et al., 1932). This observation led WADDELL to postulate the existence of another vitamin D that could be produced by the irradiation of impure cholesterol solutions (WADDELL, 1934). The WINDAUS group chemically synthesized 7-dehydrocholesterol (WINDAUS et al., 1935), and upon irradiation, produced the other major form of vitamin D, namely, vitamin D_3 (SCHENCK, 1937). Thus in 1937 the isolation and identification of the vitamin D nutritional compounds had been completed, drawing to a close this important era of vitamin D investigation. From that time forward it was assumed that vitamin D must function directly to bring about the healing of rickets, a belief that was strengthened by the early experiments of KODICEK and his colleagues in which the conclusion was reached that vitamin D was active without metabolic alteration (KODICEK, 1956). This idea, however, was later to be reversed with the introduction of modern biochemical techniques, which have now clearly demonstrated that vitamin D must be metabolically altered and in fact is converted to a hormone that then functions in calcium and phosphorus metabolism.

While the chemistry of vitamin D was being elucidated by the brilliant work of WINDAUS et al. (1932) and ASKEW et al. (1931), considerable progress was made in understanding the physiologic functions of the vitamin. Rickets itself was recognized as a disease that results from failure of the mineral of bone to be deposited in the newly forming bone centers. Thus in rapidly growing children or animals, large amounts of organic matrix of bone are elaborated, but they fail to mineralize. Although at first sight this disease might be considered a disease of the bone itself, HOWLAND and KRAMER (1921) provided evidence to the contrary. They demonstrated that the major problem with failure to mineralize bone in rachitic children was that calcium and phosphorus concentrations plasma were far below normal. They also carried out experiments in which slices of rachitic cartilage were incubated with rachitic serum and failed to calcify whereas the rachitic cartilage incubated in normal serum underwent calcification in the hypertrophic zone (SHIPLEY et al., 1925; 1926). They reasoned that vitamin D deficiency is a disease of the blood rather than one of the bone. Although these experiments raised many questions, their conclusions have been remarkably true. A low product of calcium times phosphorus has been used as a diagnostic test of rickets for many years, but nevertheless the search continued for a role for vitamin D in the mineralization process of bone, v. i.

The large amount of calcium in the feces of rachitic children led ORR and his colleagues to conclude that an important function of vitamin D is to improve gastrointestinal absorption of calcium (ORR et al., 1923). Work by others also confirmed the large fecal loss of calcium under conditions of vitamin D deficiency. However, many scientists reasoned that the increased fecal calcium might be due to failure to mineralize bone, bringing about large endogenous losses of calcium. Therefore, vitamin D might not directly improve intestinal absorption of calcium. However, the classical experiments of NICOLAYSEN conclusively demonstrated that vitamin D specifically improves intestinal absorption of calcium and that vitamin D does not influence the endogenous loss of calcium or excretion into the intestinal tract (NICOLAYSEN, 1937a, b, c). NICOLAYSEN in further classical experiments demonstrated that the intestine had the remarkable ability of improving its efficiency of absorption of calcium when there were large needs for calcium by the organism, whereas efficiency of calcium absorption was markedly suppressed under conditions of calcium sufficiency (NICOLAYSEN et al., 1953). NICOLAYSEN further found that this ability of the intestine to adapt required the presence of vitamin D, thus demonstrating another important function of the vitamin, namely, to allow the intestine to alter its efficiency of calcium absorption to meet the needs of the organism. NICOLAYSEN's classical work has been repeatedly confirmed using much more elegant techniques (WASSERMAN, 1963), and in fact the improved intestinal absorption brought about by vitamin D was demonstrated in vitro because of the classical experiments of SCHACHTER and his colleagues (SCHACHTER and ROSEN, 1959; SCHACHTER et al., 1961). Thus an important function of vitamin D is to improve intestinal absorption of calcium.

Although NICOLAYSEN suggested that vitamin D does not improve intestinal phosphate absorption (NICOLAYSEN, 1937d), the work of HARRISON and HARRISON clearly demonstrated that vitamin D plays a direct role in phosphorus metabolism, particularly in improving intestinal phosphate absorption (HARRISON and HARRISON, 1961). It is now clear that this function of vitamin D is independent of its function on calcium absorption.

The search for the role of vitamin D in mineralization caused investigators to ignore a fundamental role of vitamin D in another aspect of bone metabolism. CARLSSON and colleagues demonstrated that vitamin D, rather than functioning directly in the mineralization process, functions instead on the mobilization of calcium from the bone compartment (CARLSSON, 1952; BAUER et al., 1955). Using both radioisotopic methods and simple nutritional experiments, CARLSSON clearly demonstrated that vitamin D plays an important role in the utilization of calcium from bone to support plasma calcium concentration (CARLSSON, 1952). This function was subsequently shown to be interrelated with the effects of the parathyroid hormone on this system (HARRISON et al., 1958; RASMUSSEN et al., 1963).

Attention was also focused on the possibility that vitamin D improved renal reabsorption of calcium and phosphorus (HARRISON and HARRISON, 1941). Although current evidence suggests that vitamin D does improve renal reabsorption of calcium in concert with parathyroid hormone, it also seems clear that vitamin D does not improve renal reabsorption of phosphorus. Indeed, more recent work suggests that vitamin D may play an indirect role in phosphate excretion under conditions of hyperphosphatemia (BONJOUR and FLEISCH, 1977).

Repeatedly there have been advocates of the concept that vitamin D must function in the mineralization process. Although this may well prove to be the case, and it is certainly intellectually pleasing to consider, so far no experiment has been performed that shows clearly or conclusively that vitamin D must function somewhere in the mineralization process. In fact, all experiments to date are consistent with the idea that vitamin D improves mineralization of bone by elevating plasma calcium and phosphorus concentrations to a level that will support mineralization of newly forming bone (DELUCA, 1967; LAMM and NEUMAN, 1958). However, the idea that vitamin D might function in improving mineralization directly cannot be excluded at this time and must remain an area for continued investigation.

C. The D Vitamins and Their Precursors

It must be recognized that there is not a single vitamin D compound but that there is a family of compounds that exhibit vitamin D activity. The most important of the vitamin D compounds are vitamins D_2 and D_3 (Fig. 1), and the more important of these is vitamin D_3 or cholecalciferol. The basis for this statement is that vitamin D_3 is the vitamin produced in the skin by ultraviolet irradiation. Vitamin D_2, however, is produced by ultraviolet irradiation of the plant sterol ergosterol (Fig. 2). The photolysis reaction that converts the 5,7-diene sterols to the corresponding D vitamins, as shown in Fig. 3 has been examined intensively. It is known that 250–310 nm ultraviolet light brings about the photolytic conversion of vitamin D to the previtamin D (Havinga, 1973, Velluz and Amiard, 1949a). Further activation by light photons brings about the formation of tachysterol, a relatively unstable irradiation product, and lumisterol. The previtamin D is in thermal equilibrium with vitamin D_3 and upon heating will rapidly convert to the vitamin D structure. The equilibrium is temperature dependent, and the relative concentrations of the forms of vitamin D at

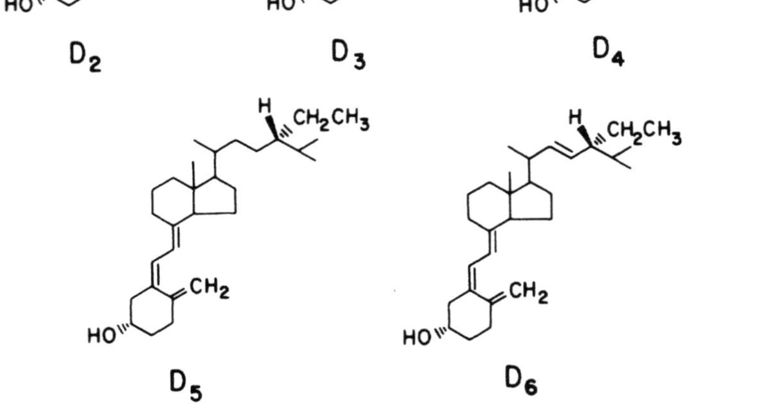

Fig. 1. Structures of the D vitamins

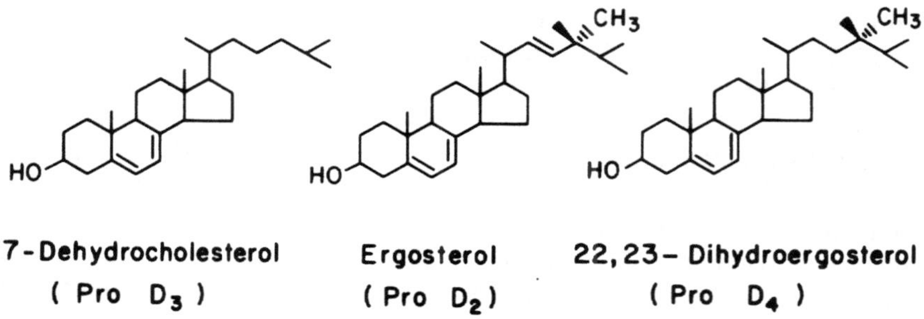

Fig. 2. The sterol precursors of the most common of the known vitamin D substances

equilibrium are a function of temperature (VELLUZ and AMIARD, 1949b; VELLUZ et al., 1949). At room temperature the conversion of the previtamin to the vitamin is slow, and even at skin temperatures it is a very slow process.

There are other forms of vitamin D known (Fig. 1) and their precursors are shown in Fig. 2. At present, the most significant of these minor forms is vitamin D_4, which was synthesized as an analog of vitamin D_2 by WINDAUS and TRAUTMAN (1937). This form of vitamin D is a chemical and biochemical curiosity and has been synthesized once again in recent years. In mammals its biological activity is only two-

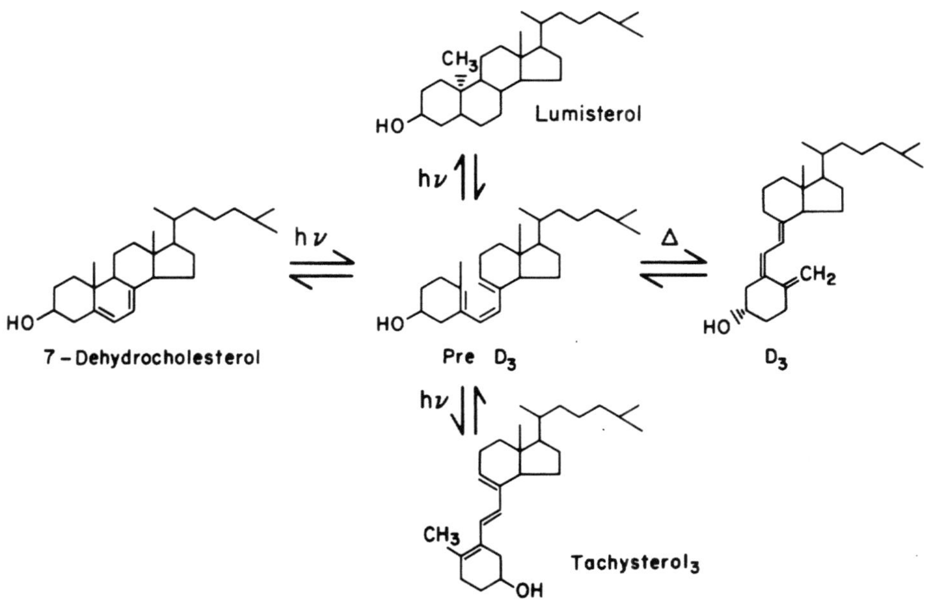

Fig. 3. Structural representation of the photolysis reaction that results in the production of vitamin D_3. Note that previtamin D_3 is the central intermediate that can be converted to either lumisterol$_3$ or tachysterol$_3$ as side-reaction products. Vitamin D_3 results from the thermally dependent equilibration of previtamin D to vitamin D_3

thirds or three-fourths that of vitamin D_2 or vitamin D_3 (WINDAUS and TRAUTMAN, 1937; DELUCA et al., 1968), whereas vitamin D_2 and vitamin D_3 are approximately equipotent. In birds, however, vitamin D_2 is one-tenth as active as vitamin D_3 in every respect (CHEN and BOSMANN, 1964). Curiously, New World monkeys show similar discrimination against the vitamin D_2 compounds (HUNT et al., 1967). It is indeed possible that in the future, subtle differences may well be found between vitamin D_2 and vitamin D_3 in other mammals as well. A basis for discrimination against the vitamin D_2 compounds in birds will be discussed later. A detailed discussion of the chemical characteristics of the D vitamins including their mass spectra, nuclear magnetic resonance spectra, etc. has been published elsewhere and interested readers are directed to those sources (HOLICK and DELUCA, 1974; DELUCA, 1978).

D. Metabolism of Vitamin D

Our understanding of the metabolism of vitamin D_3 is far from complete. However, almost all of the discussion relates to discoveries made during the past decade, and it is indeed surprising that so much information has become known in that short period. Much remains to be learned, however, concerning the nature of the excretory products of the D vitamins, the sites of inactivation as well as possible further activation.

I. Absorption of Vitamin D_3

It has been recognized since the early work of SIR EDWARD MELLANBY that vitamin D must be easily absorbed. This conclusion is well supported by work with radioactive vitamin D showing that up to 80 percent of the adminstered radioactive vitamin in oil is absorbed (NORMAN and DELUCA, 1963; KODICEK, 1960; NEVILLE and DELUCA, 1966). This 80 percent figure is probably low since some of the radioactivity appearing in the feces may well have been vitamin D that was absorbed, inactivated, and excreted. Because it is fat-soluble, vitamin D is undoubtedly absorbed as other lipid materials in which bile salts must be considered essential. This was clearly demonstrated by the work of GREAVES and SCHMIDT (1933) and more recently by SCHACHTER and colleagues (1964). Little is known concerning the mechanism of vitamin D_3 absorption, and the sites of vitamin D absorption are not agreed upon. Vitamin D in oil solutions seems to be absorbed primarily in the distal small intestine in the rat (KODICEK, 1950; NORMAN and DELUCA, 1963). SCHACHTER and his colleagues, however, found that vitamin D in alcoholic and bile salt suspensions is absorbed more rapidly in the upper small intestinal tract (SCHACHTER et al., 1964). Obviously much additional work remains to be carried out in this important area, although great care must be exercised in these studies because of the instability of the vitamin D molecule to oxidation. It seems likely that vitamin D, being a fat-soluble substance, must be absorbed with the neutral lipids, making its appearance in the lymphatic system as chylomicrons (AVIOLI et al., 1967; RIKKERS et al., 1969). Vitamin D_3 from the chylomicrons or following injection as an alcoholic solution is rapidly taken up by the liver (NORMAN and DELUCA, 1963; KODICEK, 1960; NEVILLE and DELUCA, 1966; AVIOLI et al., 1967).

II. Production of Vitamin D in the Skin

As pointed out earlier, it is known that solutions of 7-dehydrocholesterol or other 5,7-diene sterols in organic solvents undergo photolysis under the influence of ultraviolet (UV) light. This reaction obviously does not require the presence of any tissue component since it takes place in pure organic solvents. The presence of 7-dehydrocholesterol in the epidermis of skin is well recognized, and in fact it is known that 7-dehydrocholesterol can be produced in large amounts in the skin (IDLER and BAUMANN, 1952; BLOCH, 1965). More recent work has demonstrated that radioactive 7-dehydrocholesterol from the systemic circulation can make its appearance in the epidermis (HOLICK et al., 1977). It is known that uv light of the correct wavelength will penetrate the epidermis (DANIELS, 1964), and thus it is surmised that the 7-dehydrocholesterol present there will undergo photolysis to form previtamin D. This substance can then over a period of hours slowly isomerize to vitamin D_3. Because irradiation of skin induced antirachitic activity, it was assumed that vitamin D_3 was the product (DELUCA et al., 1971). More recently it has been possible to demonstrate conclusively that the antirachitic substance induced in skin by uv irradiation is truly vitamin D_3 (HOLICK et al., 1977; ESVELT et al., 1977). This substance has been isolated in pure form from the skin of rats low in vitamin D following up irradiation and identified by mass spectrometry and uv absorption spectrophotometry. There have been reports that previtamin D_3 has been isolated, although characterization of that product remains unclear (PATROVA et al., 1976). However, on the basis of the thermodynamics of previtamin D_3 formation by photolysis, there is no question that previtamin D_3 must be the intermediate and must be the major substance that appears following uv irradiation of 7-dehydrocholesterol in skin. So far, there is no clear evidence of the participation of any protein or enzyme in the catalysis of this reaction. Thus it is likely that this conversion occurs much as it does in organic solvents, i. e. not involving any protein or catalytic substance. It seems evident, therefore, that this process is probably not regulated, although regulation of the amount of 7-dehydrocholesterol by the intensity of uv light has been reported (WELLS and BAUMANN, 1954). It is also intellectually more satisfying to believe that the control of the functional metabolism of vitamin D is found further along the pathway and closer to the ultimate active form. Vitamin D_3 is tranported in the blood bound to an α-globulin (RIKKERS et al., 1969; RIKKERS and DELUCA, 1967; IMAWARI et al., 1976; HADDAD and WALGATE, 1976). Although some binding to the β-lipoproteins and to albumin has been reported, it seems clear that the primary vitamin D transport protein is the 52,000 molecular weight α-globulin. This protein has been isolated in pure form from the plasma of man (IMAWARI et al., 1976; HADDAD and WALGATE, 1976) and of rats (BOTHAM et al., 1976). It has a molecular weight of 52,000 daltons, is quite stable, and appears identical to the group-specific component isolated previously (BOUILLON et al., 1976; DAIGER et al., 1975). This protein has a binding capacity greatly in excess of the amount of vitamin D and its metabolites present in plasma, and it seems likely that it must have some other function besides transport of vitamin D molecules. Although there has been much speculation as to how much vitamin D circulates in the plasma, recently, methods have been developed in the author's laboratory using high-pressure liquid chromatography (unpublished results), which demonstrate that, normally, in man and in cows the circulating level of vitamin D_3 is about 1–2 ng/ml, below that of its major metabolite 25-hydroxyvitamin D_3 (25-OH-D_3). The transport protein in the plasma has not been studied in any detail, and it is not known how many peptide chains are present nor is anything known concerning its terminal amino acids, or amino acid sequence.

III. Storage of Vitamin D

It is known that vitamin D is stored to a considerable extent. For example, it was shown that injection of vitamin D in large doses resulted in its detection in livers six months later (HEYMANN, 1937). The initial accumulation of radioactive vitamin D in the liver led KODICEK to conclude that the liver is the major storage organ for the vitamin (KODICEK, 1956; BLUMBERG et al., 1960). The presence of significant amounts of vitamin D in the liver also supported this belief. However, QUARTERMAN questioned whether the liver can be considered a storage organ of vitamin D (QUARTERMAN, 1964). A more definitive series of experiments by ROSENSTREICH et al. (1971) have demonstrated that the vitamin is stored primarily in the fat depots rather than specifically in the liver, as was once believed. Depletion of animals dosed with vitamin D is indeed a long process, primarily because it depends upon the turnover of lipid depots, which probably takes considerable time. In animals or man given large doses of vitamin D, depletion is likely to require not months but years. The half-life of vitamin D in the plasma appears to be short and has been estimated to be 22 h (AVIOLI et al., 1967). However, it is likely that the lifetime of vitamin D in the plasma is even shorter, whereas in the tissues and body, it must be an extremely long period, probably measured in weeks if not months. Unfortunately, accurate data are not available on this particular aspect of vitamin D storage and turnover.

IV. Role of the Liver in Production of 25-Hydroxyvitamin D_3 (Fig. 4)

Vitamin D that reaches the blood compartment from all sources is rapidly cleared by the liver. In fact, PONCHON and DELUCA (1969a) demonstrated that within 60 min the vitamin D in the plasma is cleared and accumulates in the liver. Radioactivity from radioactive vitamin D then begins to appear in the plasma 3–4 h postinjection. The radioactivity appearing in the plasma is found primarily as its major metabolite, 25-OH-D_3 (PONCHON and DELUCA, 1969a). These experiments plus hepatectomy studies led to the conclusion that the liver is the major but not sole site of 25-hydroxylation of vitamin D in mammals (PONCHON et al., 1969; OLSON et al., 1976). In birds, TUCKER et al. (1973) demonstrated that 25-OH-D_3 could be produced by intestinal and kidney homogenates. Although work in the author's laboratory did not confirm the presence of 25-hydroxylation in kidney tissue, 25-hydroxylation in intestinal tissue taken from birds was confirmed (BHATTACHARYYA and DELUCA, 1974a). However, no 25-hydroxylation could be found in intestinal preparations from rats (HOLICK et al., 1976a). Furthermore, a detailed examination of the hepatectomized rat led to the conclusion that the major site of 25-hydroxylation is the liver (OLSON et al., 1976). The vitamin D_3 25-hydroxylase is found primarily in the microsomal fraction (BHATTACHARYYA and DELUCA, 1974b). This system requires NADPH, molecular oxygen, magnesium ions, and the cytosolic fraction. The reason for the cytosolic requirement remains unknown, although it may be that this substance is necessary to protect the labile cis-triene structure of the D vitamin from oxidative degradation or that the cytosolic protein may be required to transport

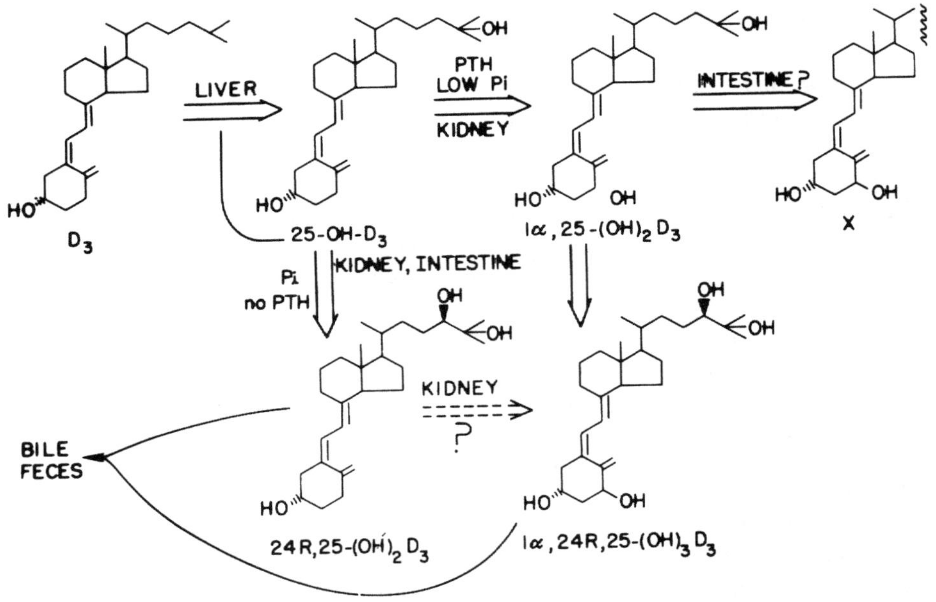

Fig. 4. The known metabolic pathways of vitamin D metabolism to its active hormone 1,25-$(OH)_2D_3$. Note that 24-hydroxylation of both the active hormone 1,25-$(OH)_2D_3$ and its precursor 25-OH-D_3 is known to occur in kidney and intestine. In addition, 1,25-$(OH)_2D_3$ undergoes side-chain oxidative cleavage to yield an unknown metabolite X

vitamin D to the hydroxylation sites in the microsomes or to transport the 25-OH-D_3 product from the microsomes. This problem has not yet been solved. Little is known concerning the nature of the 25-hydroxylase. Work has been completed with oxygen-18, which demonstrates that it is, in fact, a mixed function monooxygenase (MADHOK et al., unpublished work). Spectral evidence for the binding of vitamin D and 25-OH-D_3 to microsomal P450 has been obtained, but its meaning remains unknown since products of microsomal reactions have not yet been identified other than 25-OH-D_3 (CINTI et al., 1976; GHAZARIAN et al., 1977). However, carbon monoxide does inhibit the production of 25-OH-D_3 from vitamin D_3 (MADHOK and DELUCA, unpublished results), although this possibility has not been exhaustively examined. Cytochrome P450 inhibitors do block 25-hydroxylation of vitamin D while peroxidation inhibitors such as diphenylparaphenylene diamine or electron transport inhibitors do not (HORSTING, 1970). Thus, although it is likely that 25-hydroxylase is a mixed function monooxygenase, little definitive work is yet available on this particular enzyme.

The 25-OH-D_3 (BLUNT et al., 1968a), which is formed in the liver, is more active than vitamin D_3, it is 2–5 times more active than the parent vitamin in all the systems known to be responsive to vitamin D (BLUNT et al., 1968a; TANAKA et al., 1973a). The structure of 25-OH-D_3 was unequiviocally determined in 1968 (BLUNT et al., 1968a), followed by chemical synthesis in 1969 (BLUNT and DELUCA, 1969) to establish firmly its identity. Although 25-OH-D_3 in pharmacologic amounts is known to act on the target organs of vitamin D (PAVLOVITCH et al., 1973), it is now clear that at physiologic concentrations it is not active and must be converted further to its hormonal form (BOYLE et al., 1972a; HOLICK et al., 1972a). 25-OH-D_3 does not accumulate in the liver and is transported on the 52,000 molecular weight vitamin D transport protein to the kidney where it undergoes further modification. 25-OH-D_3 is the major circulating form of the vitamin, being present at 25–35 ng/ml in normal, well-nourished adults and children (HADDAD and STAMP, 1974; EISMAN et al., 1977; ARNAUD et al., 1977). Lower figures have been found in Canada, Britain, and in the United States, especially in the springtime following a winter of presumably low incidence of uv irradiation (STAMP and ROUND, 1974; LESTER et al., 1977; ELLIS et al., 1977). The dissociation constant of 25-OH-D_3 and the transport protein is 2×10^{-9} M, indicating that it is indeed tightly bound (HADDAD and BIRGE, 1975; MELLON and DELUCA, unpublished results). It seems clear that the transport protein from different species may show different dissociation constants for 25-OH-D_3. Thus it might appear that in birds the dissociation constant may be one or two orders of magnitude larger than in the rat.

How the 25-OH-D_3 is transferred to the kidney remains unknown. In the kidney, the 25-OH-D_3 undergoes one of two hydroxylations. As will be discussed in the regulation of vitamin D metabolism, if there is a need for calcium, as signaled by high parathyroid hormone levels, or a need for phosphorus, as signaled by hypophosphatemia, or other factors that signal abnormal calcium requirements, 25-OH-D_3 is hydroxylated on carbon 1 to yield 1,25-dihydroxyvitamin D_3 [1,25-$(OH)_2D_3$]. The identity of this hormonal form of vitamin D was unequivocally established in 1970–1971 by mass spectrometry of the product isolated in pure form from the target organ of intestine and by specific chemical reactions carried out on this product followed by mass spectrometry (HOLICK et al., 1971a, b). This work allowed the conclusion that the structure was 1,25-$(OH)_2D_3$. Chemical synthesis of 1α,25-$(OH)_2D_3$, achieved in 1972 (SEMMLER et al., 1972), permitted the confident conclusion that the active hormone is probably 1α,25-$(OH)_2D_3$. However, because the 1β,25-$(OH)_2D_3$ compound had not been synthesized, it was not possible to exclude that the natural product might be 1β,25-$(OH)_2D_3$. More recently, we have completed chemical synthesis of 1β,25-$(OH)_2D_3$ (PAAREN et al., 1978), and demonstrated both biologically and chromatographically that it is different from the natural product. This conclusively demonstrates that the natural product is indeed 1α,25-$(OH)_2D_3$.

The 25-OH-D_3-1α-hydroxylase is found exclusively in the kidney inasmuch as nephrectomy prevents in vivo production of this metabolite from 25-OH-D_3 (FRASER and KODICEK, 1970; GRAY et al., 1971; NORMAN et al., 1971). Furthermore, this enzyme is found exclusively in the mitochondrial fraction in birds, though its exact submitochondrial location is not yet known (FRASER and KODICEK, 1970; GRAY et al., 1972). Experiments with oxygen-18 have clearly demonstrated that this enzyme is a mixed-function monooxygenase (GHAZARIAN et al., 1973). In addition, it is now known that this mixed-function monooxygenase is supported by NADPH, molecular oxygen, and magnesium ions (GHAZARIAN and DELUCA, 1974). However, the dependence on NADPH could only be demonstrated when mitochondria were sufficiently swollen or ruptured to permit entry of NADPH. Thus calcium-swollen mitochondria will carry out hydroxylation provided that NADPH is generated by an exogenous NADPH-generating system. When hydroxylation in calcium-swollen mitochondria is supported by NADPH from external sources, the hydroxylation of 25-OH-D_3 is not dependent on oxidative phosphorylation and thus is not blocked by inhibitors such as cyanide, dinitrophenol, and oligomycin (GHAZARIAN and DELUCA, 1974). On the other hand, if the mitochondria are maintained intact, the 1-hydroxylase must be supported by a Krebs cycle substrate such as malate, succinate, etc. When the reaction is supported in this manner, uncouplers of oxidative phosphorylation or electron transport inhibitors block the reaction. It therefore appears that in intact mitochondria internally generated NADPH is required which is dependent upon energy-linked transhydrogenation and/or reversal of electron transport. The 25-OH-D_3-1-hydroxylase has a very specific requirement for the intact vitamin D molecule with a 25-hydroxy group (GRAY et al., 1972; TANAKA et al., 1976a). Thus neither 24-OH-D_3 nor vitamin D_3 itself can serve as a substrate for this enzyme (TANAKA et al., 1976a). Of special interest is the fact that dihydrotachesterol that has the A ring rotated and the 10–19 double bond system reduced, cannot undergo 1α-hydroxylation (HALLICK and DELUCA, 1971). In addition, the 1α-hydroxylase will only slowly insert a 1-hydroxyl on a compound that has a 24(*S*),25-dihydroxy function (TANAKA et al., 1976a). As will be discussed later, this is the basis for discrimination against the 24S hydroxyl of 24,25-dihydroxyvitamin D_3 [24,25-$(OH)_2D_3$]. A great deal of work has been expended in deciphering the enzymology of the 1-hydroxylase system of rachitic chick kidney mitochondria. Thus inhibitors of cytochrome P450-dependent reactions have been shown to block the 1-hydroxylation of 25-OH-D_3 in vitro. Carbon monoxide mixtures inhibit the reaction and this inhibition can be relieved by white light (GHAZARIAN and DELUCA, 1974) or more specifically by light of 450 nm wavelength (HENRY and NORMAN, 1974). In addition, metyrapone and glutethimide, inhibitors of the P450 reactions, inhibit 1-hydroxylase (GHAZARIAN et al., 1974). Additional evidence has been brought forth to demonstrate that mitochondria from rachitic chicks contain a cytochrome P450 that is reducible by the addition of malate or other Krebs cycle substrates, thereby eliminating the possibility that the P450 is a microsomal contaminant. The cytochrome P450 has been solubilized from rachitic chick mitochondria and when incubated together with beef adrenal ferredoxin, beef adrenal ferredoxin reductase, and NADPH, 1-hydroxylation of 25-OH-D_3 can be demonstrated in vitro (GHAZARIAN et al., 1974). The iron-sulfur protein from chick kidney mitochondria has now been isolated in pure form (PEDERSEN et al., 1976; YOON and DELUCA, unpublished results) and when combined with beef adrenal ferredoxin reductase and cytochrome P450 from rachitic chick kidney mitochondria, 1α-hydroxylation of 25-OH-D_3 is very rapid, yielding only one product, 1,25-$(OH)_2D_3$. Based on these experiments it is clear that the mechanism of the 25-OH-D_3-1-

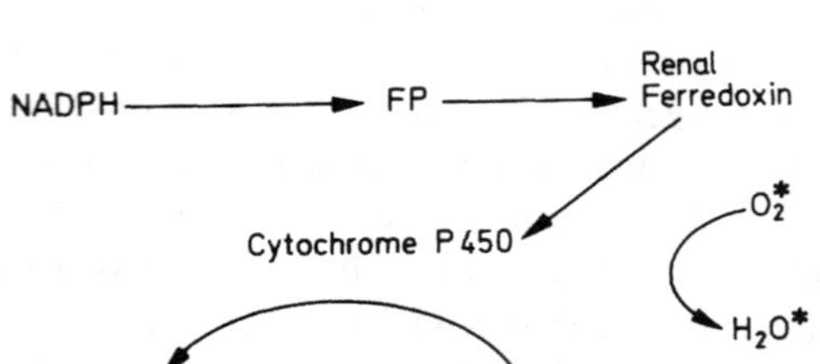

Fig. 5. A molecular mechanism of hydroxylation of 25-OH-D_3 to 1α,25-$(OH)_2D_3$ in chick renal mitochondria. Note that the enzymatic machinery responsible for this conversion is similar to the steroidogenesis system of the adrenals

hydroxylation reaction is as depicted in Fig. 5. This reaction is analogous to the steroidogenesis reactions that occur in the adrenal gland involving a similar enzymologic mechanism (SIH, 1969). As will be demonstrated in the regulation section, the parallel between the 1α-hydroxylase and the adrenal steroidogenesis system is remarkable.

The 1,25-$(OH)_2D_3$ formed in the kidney is then transported via the 52,000 molecular weight plasma protein to the target tissues of intestine, bone, and elsewhere in the kidney where it functions on calcium and phosphorus transport reactions. To demonstrate the essentiality of the 1-hydroxylation reaction to the function of vitamin D at physiologic concentrations, the experiments rely heavily on the fact that the kidney is the sole site of production of 1,25-$(OH)_2D_3$ (FRASER and KODICEK, 1970; GRAY et al., 1971). Thus in vitamin D-deficient, nephrectomized animals physiologic amounts of 25-OH-D_3 do not stimulate intestinal calcium transport (BOYLE et al., 1972a), phosphate transport (CHEN et al., 1974), or mobilize calcium from bone. On the other hand, the same animals respond equally well to 1,25-$(OH)_2D_3$ whether kidneys are present or not. These experiments demonstrate clearly that 1,25-$(OH)_2D_3$ or a further metabolite is the metabolically active form of the vitamin in carrying out its functions in the intestine and bone and that 25-OH-D_3 and vitamin D_3 do not function at physiologic concentrations in these target organs.

V. Metabolism of 25-Hydroxyvitamin D_3 to 24,25-Dihydroxyvitamin D_3

Following the isolation and identification of 25-OH-D_3 in 1968 (BLUNT et al., 1968a), an intense interest developed in the metabolism of vitamin D_3 and 25-OH-D_3 to its active metabolites. It soon became clear that a metabolite more polar than 25-OH-D_3 appeared in the profiles of sterol extracted from intestines of rachitic rats (PONCHON and DELUCA, 1969b; DELUCA, 1970) or chicks (LAWSON et al., 1969; HAUSSLER et al., 1968) given radioactive vitamin D_3. Reports on the biological activity of this more polar metabolite peak from silicic acid columns varied. At least some biological activity could be found, however, in peak V as described in this laboratory, peak 4B from HAUSSLER and NORMAN, and peak P from KODICEK and his colleagues. This led to the isolation and identification of two metabolites from the plasma of pigs given large amounts of vitamin D. The first of these metabolites was initially identified as 21,25-dihydroxyvitamin D_3 [21,25-$(OH)_2D_3$] (SUDA et al., 1970a). This compound was left unattended while continuing investigations led to the isolation and identification of 1,25-$(OH)_2D_3$ (HOLICK et al., 1971a, b). Following the identification of 1,25-$(OH)_2D_3$, BOYLE and colleagues demonstrated that in animals given vitamin D and sufficient amounts of calcium, 1,25-$(OH)_2D_3$ was not the major product of 25-OH-D_3 but instead another product somewhat less polar than 1,25-$(OH)_2D_3$ on Sephadex LH-20 columns was noted (BOYLE et al., 1971; 1972b). BOYLE studied this compound more thoroughly and found that it indeed possessed biological activity but that its biological activity required the presence of the kidney (BOYLE et al., 1973). This compound appeared to have biological activity almost equivalent to that of 25-OH-D_3 in the rat. This led to the isolation and identification of this metabolite from in vitro incubations of kidney preparations from animals given high calcium diets and vitamin D_3 (HOLICK et al., 1972b). This substance was identified as 24,25-$(OH)_2D_3$ and appeared to migrate in exactly the same position as the previously isolated 21,25-$(OH)_2D_3$. A reexamination of 21,25-$(OH)_2D_3$ resulted in a revision of that identification (HOLICK et al., 1972b). The marked biological activity of this compound in mammals (HOLICK et al., 1972b) led to the chemical synthesis of the two possible isomers of this compound by two different research groups. Thus the Hoffmann-LaRoche chemists under the direction of Milan Uskokovic (PARTRIDGE et al., 1976) and the Tokyo Institute of Technology chemists under the direction of Professor Nobuo IKEKAWA (SEKI et al., 1975) chemically synthesized the S and R epimers of the 24-hydroxy compounds. Using the synthetic compounds, TANAKA et al. (1975a) demonstrated clearly that the natural product possesses the 24R configuration, whereas the S configuration was a synthetic curiosity. The 24R-hydroxyvitamin D_3 (24R-OH-D_3) and 24R,25-$(OH)_2D_3$ both had marked biological activity in vitamin D-deficient rats in every respect, whereas the S configuration showed markedly little biological activity (BORIS et al., 1977; HENRY et al., 1976; TANAKA et al., 1975a). Chemical synthesis of tritium-labeled 24S and 24R-OH-D_3 and its study in rats demonstrated that both compounds are rapidly converted to the 25-hydroxy derivative but that only the 24R,25-$(OH)_2D_3$ is converted further to the 1,24R,25-trihydroxyvitamin D_3 [1,24R,25-$(OH)_3D_3$], which is biologically active and will be discussed later (TANAKA et al., 1976a). In the bird 24R,25-$(OH)_2D_3$ has little biological activity, which contrasts sharply with observations in the rat (HENRY et al., 1976; HOLICK et al., 1976b). This led HOLICK et al. (1976b) to suggest that substitution on the carbon 24 might render the molecule similar to vitamin D_2, which leads to discrimination against that compound by birds. HOLICK et al. reasoned that on this basis the 24R,25-$(OH)_2D_3$ may be an initial inactivation product. An investigation into the enzymology of the 24-hydroxylase in kidney tissue has demonstrated it to be a mitochondrial enzyme (KNUTSON and DELUCA, 1974) and with oxygen 18 it has been found to be a mixed-function monooxygenase (MADHOK et al., 1977). It is supported in intact mitochondria by internally generated NADPH, analogous to the 1-hydroxylase system, and is supported in swollen mitochondria by externally generated NADPH (KNUTSON and DELUCA, 1974). So far the details of the components of this hydroxylase have not been elucidated. However, it is not as sensitive to carbon monoxide–oxygen mixtures as is the 1-hydroxylase. Thus far, therefore, it is uncertain whether the 24-hydroxylase is in fact a cytochrome P450 reaction.

In contrast to the 1-hydroxylase, nephrectomy does not completely eliminate 24-hydroxylation of 25-OH-D_3 (BOYLE et al., 1973; KUMAR and DELUCA, 1978). Therefore, the kidney is not the sole site of 24-hydroxylation; in fact more recent work has demonstrated the existence of a 24-hydroxylase in intestinal tissue (KUMAR and DELUCA, 1978), and another report suggests its presence in cartilage tissue (GARABEDIAN et al., 1977). The 24-hydroxylase requires that a vitamin D molecule have a 25-hydroxyl function. It is unknown whether 24-hydroxylation occurs on dihydrotachysterol or 5,6-trans-25-OH-D_3. Therefore, it is uncertain whether the 24-hydroxylase requires an intact cis-triene structure and an appropriate stereochemical arrangement for the ring A portion of the vitamin D molecule.

The biological importance of 24-hydroxylation remains unknown. In birds 24-hydroxylation causes reduction in biological activity whereas in the rat 24R-hydroxylation does not enhance the activity and may only slightly reduce it. Based on these observations it is believed that 24-hydroxylation is the initial event in inactivation of the vitamin D molecule. The 24-hydroxylase appears to be a regulated enzyme and when the 1-hydroxylase is suppressed, the 24-hydroxylase is generally elevated. Furthermore, as will be shown below, the 24-hydroxylase appears to be induced or at least enhanced by 1,25-$(OH)_2D_3$. Monkey kidney cells grown in culture will 24-hydroxylate 25-OH-D_3 (JUAN and DELUCA, 1977). In this system high ambient calcium concentrations and additions of 1,25-$(OH)_2D_3$ markedly enhance the 24-hydroxylase whereas parathyroid hormone suppresses the 24-hydroxylase. Considerable work has been expended in attempting to demonstrate a special function for this metabolite of vitamin D. Thus reports have appeared that the 24,25-$(OH)_2D_3$ has a special function in calcification (BORDIER et al., 1977), in suppression of parathyroid hormone secretion (HENRY, 1977), and in intestinal calcium absorption (KANIS et al., 1975). These ideas remain highly controversial and certainly not established at the present time.

VI. Production of 1,24,25-Trihydroxyvitamin D_3

As was discussed in the previous section, the biological activity of 24,25-$(OH)_2D_3$ can only be found in animals retaining their kidneys. This led to the suggestion by BOYLE et al. (1973) that 24,25-$(OH)_2D_3$ must be converted to 1,24,25-$(OH)_3D_3$ before it is effective in stimulating intestinal calcium transport or in stimulating the mobilization of calcium from bone. When 24,25-$(OH)_2D_3$ was incubated with renal homogenates taken from rachitic chickens, a metabolite was isolated in pure form and its structure was unequivocally determined as 1,24,25-$(OH)_3D_3$ (HOLICK et al., 1973a). This compound proved to be more active than 24,25-$(OH)_2D_3$ but less active than 1,25-$(OH)_2D_3$ (HOLICK et al., 1973a; CASTILLO et al., 1978). In fact, it elicits less than half the activity of 1,25-$(OH)_2D_3$ in stimulating intestinal calcium transport and is about one-tenth as active in the mobilization of calcium from bone, the elevation of serum phosphorus concentration, and in the mineralization of bone. It has a time course of response similar to that of 1,25-$(OH)_2D_3$ (CASTILLO et al., 1978). Thus its lesser activity and its time course of action suggest that it has no remarkable and unexpected activity. It therefore seems probable that 24-hydroxylation of 1,25-$(OH)_2D_3$ is an inactivation process. The 1,24,25-$(OH)_3D_3$ has been synthesized by USKOKOVIC and his colleagues at Hoffmann-LaRoche (PARTRIDGE et al., 1977) and also by IKEKAWA and his colleagues in Tokyo (IKEKAWA et al., 1975). Using the two isomers from these groups, TANAKA et al. (1977) demonstrated that the natural product is in fact 1,24R,25-$(OH)_3D_3$. In any case, the S and R isomers of this compound, in contrast to the 24,25-$(OH)_2D_3$ compounds, have equal biological activity in vivo. Thus the discrimination against the S hydroxyl occurs only at the 1-hydroxylation stage.

As will be discussed later, rachitic chickens or rats do not carry out 24-hydroxylation of 25-OH-D_3 or of 1,25-$(OH)_2D_3$ (TANAKA et al., 1975b). However, if these animals are injected with nonradioactive 1,25-$(OH)_2D_3$, the 24-hydroxylase appears. Thus one of the functions of 1,25-$(OH)_2D_3$ is probably the induction of the 24-hydroxylase enzyme. This enzyme in turn will act on 1,25-$(OH)_2D_3$ to produce 1,24,25-$(OH)_3D_3$ (TANAKA et al., 1977). This conversion is not prevented by nephrectomy (TANAKA et al., 1977), and an investigation of this problem has revealed that the intestine is a major site of 24-hydroxylation of 1,25-$(OH)_2D_3$ (KUMAR and DELUCA, 1978). Intestinal homogenates will also 24-hydroxylate 25-OH-D_3, although its activity appears to be greater on 1,25-$(OH)_2D_3$ (KUMAR and DELUCA, 1978). Thus physiologically, 1,24,25-$(OH)_3D_3$ appears to originate from the 24-hydroxylation of 1,25-$(OH)_2D_3$. Inasmuch as animals that have high levels of 24-hydroxylation usually have little or no 1-hydroxylation activity, it seems that the major route of origin of the 1,24,25-$(OH)_3D_3$ is induction of 24-hydroxylase by 1,25$(OH)_2D_3$, which in turn brings about 24-hydroxylation of 1,25-$(OH)_2D_3$. Little is known concerning the nature of the intestinal 24-hydroxylase, that was only discovered in the past few months. However, at the present time, subject to change upon further available information, it can be tentatively accepted that 24-hydroxylation of 1,25-$(OH)_2D_3$ is an initial event in the inactivation of this extremely potent molecule.

VII. Other Metabolites of Vitamin D_3

Besides 24,25-$(OH)_2D_3$, another dihydroxyvitamin D_3 metabolite has been isolated from the plasma of pigs and identified as 25,26-dihydroxyvitamin D_3 [25,26-$(OH)_2D_3$] (SUDA et al., 1970b). The site of biogenesis of this form of vitamin D is unknown and it does appear in the plasma of man (MAWER, 1977) as well as animals (SUDA et al., 1970b). Its biological activity is less than that of 25-OH-D_3 and its activity appears to be predominantly intestinal (SUDA et al., 1970b). Since nephrectomy prevents its activity (LAM et al., 1975) it is likely that it must be converted to 1,25,26-trihydroxyvitamin D_3 before it is active. Its exact role is presently unknown, although its rather small activity suggests that it is not a further activation form of vitamin D_3.

It is probable that many metabolites of vitamin D will be demonstrated in the next several years. Almost all experiments leading to the discovery of the current array of vitamin D metabolites have followed the injection of radioactive vitamin D_3 as a single dose to rachitic animals. This has led to the appearance, in the metabolite profiles, of the compounds that are believed to carry out the function of the vitamin. More recently we have carried out experiments in which radioactive vitamin D has been administered daily for a period of 1–2 weeks (RIBOVICH and DELUCA, 1978a). This has led to the discovery of a number of new metabolites of vitamin D, both nonpolar and polar, that have yet to be identified. Whether any of these will have important functions or whether they represent biochemical curiosities or inactivation products remains to be seen. However, Fig. 6 illustrates a Sephadex LH-20 column profile taken from rats given daily doses of radioactive vitamin D for a period of two weeks. A number of new metabolites can be observed, and many of the known metabolite peaks, upon subfractionation using high-pressure liquid chromatography, reveal still other metabolites. This profile illustrates that the identification of vitamin D metabolites is not yet complete, nor can one feel secure when measuring plasma levels of metabolites of vitamin D with nonspecific detection methods. It is likely that some of the unknown metabolites may interfere with such nonspecific binding substances as plasma transport protein or even cytosolic receptor proteins. In carrying

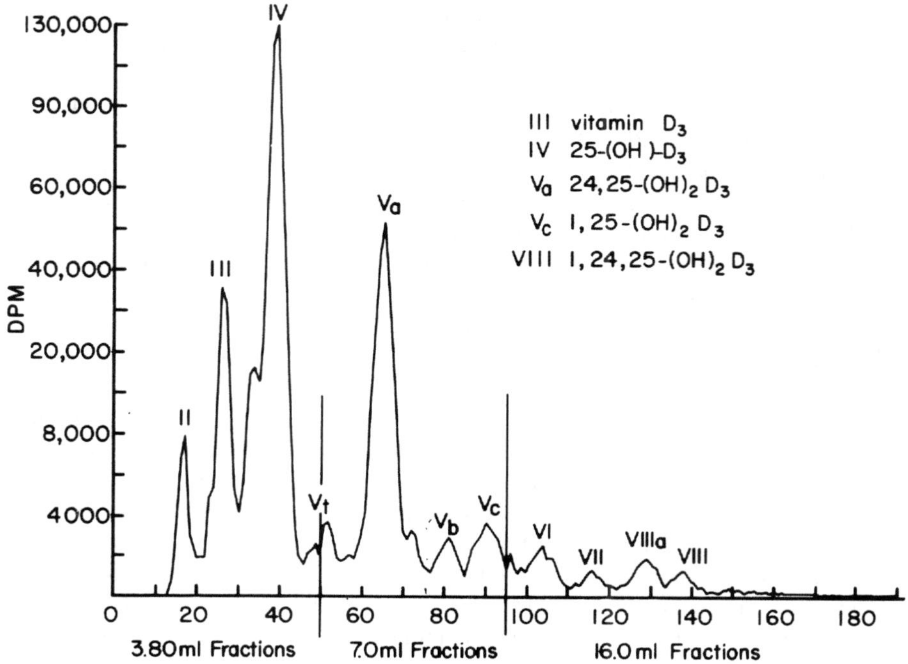

Fig. 6. Sephadex LH-20 chromatographic separation of metabolites of vitamin D that are generated in animals given daily doses of vitamin [1,2-^{3}H]D_3. Tritium-labeled vitamin D_3 was administered daily for a period of 14 days and the plasma was extracted and chromatographed on Sephadex LH-20 to reveal the metabolites indicated. Those metabolites that were positively identified are listed; the others remain as unknown compounds

out determinations of vitamin D metabolites in plasma, it is indeed extremely important to use the highest resolution chromatography available to be sure that the correct metabolite is being measured exclusively.

VIII. Metabolism of Vitamin D_2 and Dihydrotachysterols

As might be expected, vitamin D_2 is metabolized in an analogous manner to vitamin D_3 (Jones et al., 1976a). Thus 25-OH-D_2 has been isolated in pure form and its structure identified (Suda et al., 1969). It has been chemically synthesized by Campbell and Babcock at the Upjohn Company to confirm the structure identified by Suda et al. (1969). The 25-OH-D_2 is also further converted by the kidney system to 1,25-$(OH)_2D_2$, which was isolated in pure form and its structure was unequivocally identified (Jones et al., 1975). It seems likely that 25-OH-D_2 is converted to 24,25-$(OH)_2D_2$, although structural identification of this metabolite has not yet been completed. The hydroxylases that act on the vitamin D_3 series have been shown to act on vitamin D_2 compounds as well (Jones et al., 1976a). Thus the liver possesses vitamin D_2-25-hydroxylase; kidney mitochondria possess both the 1α-hydroxylase and the supposed 24R-hydroxylase. Other than this little work has been carried out with the vitamin D_2 compounds either in man or in animals primarily because of the lack of availability of the labeled material.

As pointed out earlier, New World monkeys (HUNT et al., 1967) and avian species (CHEN and BOSMANN, 1964) do not utilize vitamin D_2 as well as they do vitamin D_3. In fact estimates of biological activity in birds for vitamin D_2 is about one-tenth that of vitamin D_3 (CHEN and BOSMANN, 1964). With the discovery of the vitamin D metabolites, it was assumed that a step in the metabolic system might be responsible for the discrimination. However, JONES et al. (1976a) clearly showed that the chick liver systems hydroxylate vitamin D_2 and vitamin D_3 equally well and that the kidney systems also do not discriminate against the vitamin D_2 molecule, producing 1,25-$(OH)_2D_2$ and 1,25-$(OH)_2D_3$ in equal rates and quantities. In addition, 24-hydroxylase appears to produce equal amounts of product whether 25-OH-D_3 is used or whether 25-OH-D_2 is used, although the product has not yet been unequivocally identified. In support of this concept, JONES et al. (1976b) demonstrated that 1,25-$(OH)_2D_2$ and 25-OH-D_2 show one-tenth the activity in birds of their respective vitamin D_3 analogs. Therefore, birds discriminate against the metabolites of vitamin D_2 as well as against the vitamin D_2 molecule. This has led to the belief that birds discriminate against vitamin D_2 by rapidly metabolizing vitamin D_2 and its metabolites to excretion products. Evidence for this was obtained by IMRIE et al. (1967) with radioactive vitamin D_2 whereby it was demonstrated in birds that it is rapidly metabolized and excreted via the bile into the feces. Thus it appears that the basis for discrimination against vitamin D_2 is rapid inactivation of these molecules, presumably in the liver, although clear evidence for this has not yet been obtained. However, in mammals it can be assumed at present that vitamin D_2 undergoes the same sequential changes as vitamin D_3.

Dihydrotachysterol$_2$ was originally discovered as a product that resulted from attempts to stabilize the vitamin D compounds (von WERDER, 1939). Thus an active reduction product was obtained that was effective against hypocalcemic tetany. This led to the term antitetanic compound number 10 (AT-10). The dihydrotachysterols are reduction products in which the A ring of vitamin D_3 is rotated 180° and the C-10,19 double bond is hydrogenated as shown in Fig. 7. The exact configuration of the methyl group remains unknown and is the subject of chemical investigation by

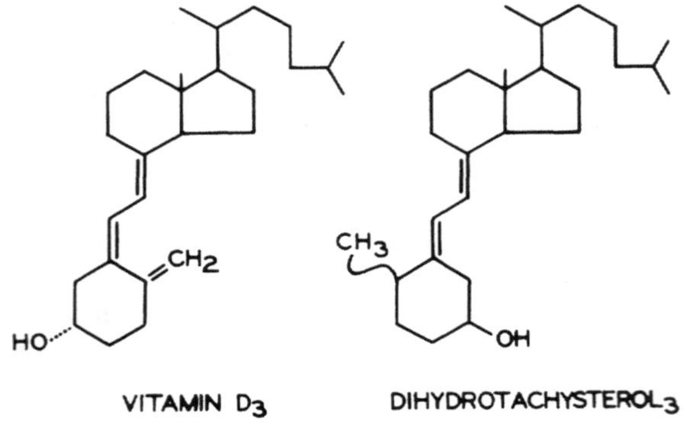

Fig. 7. The structure of dihydrotachysterol$_3$ as compared to that of vitamin D_3

two or three different groups at the present time. Dihydrotachysterol is clearly an analog of vitamin D, and it was in fact surprising that this compound should have very low antirachitic activity when given in small amounts to rachitic rats but that it possessed superior hypercalcemic activity when given in pharmacologic amounts (ALBRIGHT et al., 1938). HALLICK studied metabolism of dihydrotachysterol$_3$ and found it to be 25-hydroxylated rapidly by the liver in vivo and in vitro (HALLICK and DELUCA, 1971). 25-Hydroxydihydrotachysterol$_3$ does not serve as a substrate for the 25-OH-D_3-1-hydroxylase (TANAKA et al., 1977; HALLICK and DELUCA, 1972) and no evidence for 1,25-dihydroxydihydrotachysterol has yet been obtained. In any case, the rotation of the vitamin D A ring 180° places the 3β-hydroxyl in the position normally occupied by 1α-hydroxy of 1α,25-$(OH)_2D_3$ (HALLICK and DELUCA, 1971; 1972). Thus this compound should not require 1-hydroxylation before it is active on intestine and bone, and in fact these compounds are active in the absence of kidneys (HALLICK and DELUCA, 1971; 1972; HARRISON and HARRISON, 1971), which supports the contention that they do not require 1-hydroxylation. It is on this basis that they are successful pharmacologic agents in causing hypercalcemia or in correcting hypocalcemia. Their poor mineralization activity (SUDA et al., 1970c) (being 1/450 that of vitamin D) indicates that they are poor substances to be used when the healing of rickets or osteomalacia is required. As will be pointed out in the next section, hydroxylation of dihydrotachysterol to 25-hydroxydihydrotachysterol is not suppressed by large amounts of vitamin D or dihydrotachysterol$_3$, which also accounts for its being successful as a pharmacologic replacement for 1,25-$(OH)_2D_3$. Its further metabolism is not known at the present time, however.

Finally, some mention should be made of 5,6-trans-vitamin D_3 and isotachysterol$_3$. These compounds also have rotation of the 5,6-double bond, placing the 3β-hydroxyl in the approximate position occupied by the 1-hydroxyl of 1,25-$(OH)_2D_3$ (HOLICK et al., 1972c, d). It does not, however, have a reduced C-10,19 methylene function. These compounds are also effective in the absence of kidneys, and they are also believed to be 25-hydroxylated (LAWSON and BELL, 1974). However, their activity is also much less than that of D_3 at physiologic amounts, but it is probable that at pharmacologic amounts they would be more active than vitamin D_3. Because chemical synthesis of 1,25-$(OH)_2D_3$ and 1α-OH-D_3 has been completed, the dihydrotachysterols and transp. compounds will likely diminish in importance as therapeutic agents.

E. Regulation of Vitamin D Metabolism: The Kidney as an Endocrine Organ

I. Regulation of 25-Hydroxyvitamin D_3 Production

By biological assay it was learned prior to the isolation and identification of 25-OH-D_3 that its production (then termed peak IV) could be increased by increasing to high levels the dosage of vitamin D given to pigs (BLUNT et al., 1968a). By increasing the dietary intake of vitamin D from 90 units of antirachitic activity per pound to 250,000 units per pound of feed, the amount of circulating peak IV metabolite could be increased from 1 unit/ml to 12 units/ml. However, it is self-evident that the increase in 25-OH-D_3 production was not linearly related to the dose. Following isolation and identification of the vitamin D metabolite, it was learned that the liver is the site of 25-hydroxylation. When 25-hydroxylation was measured in vitro, no activity could be found in animals given normal levels of vitamin D whereas those on low vitamin D intakes had demonstrable activity in their liver homogenates (BHATTACHARYYA and DELUCA, 1973). Vitamin D-deficient animals had significant levels of 25-hydroxylase activity whereas those animals predosed with as little as 250 ng of vitamin D_3 6–12 h before had their 25-hydroxylase suppressed. The suppression and release of 25-hydroxylase activity were related to both dose of vitamin D and time after dose. The larger the dose the longer the period required before the 25-hydroxylase activity became measurable (BHATTACHARYYA and DELUCA, 1973). This led to the suggestion that 25-hydroxylase activity is feedback regulated by the hepatic level of 25-OH-D_3 itself. The mechanism of this suppression remains unknown, and it is possible that the suppression is merely product inhibition; on the other hand, it appears as though more is involved, such as allosteric inactivation of the 25-hydroxylase. Of great interest was the finding that dihydrotachysterol$_3$-25-hydroxylation was not suppressed either by predosage with vitamin D or with dihydrotachysterol$_3$ itself (BHATTACHARYYA and DELUCA, 1973). Similarly, the circulating level of 25-hydroxydihydrotachysterol$_3$ could be shown to increase almost with dosage of this form of vitamin D (BHATTACHARYYA and DELUCA, 1973). It therefore appeared as though two mechanisms of 25-hydroxylation may be involved: one which operates at physiologic doses of vitamin D_3 and the other which operates on sterols nonspecifically, including vitamin D at high concentrations. Nevertheless, it is evident that the suppression of 25-hydroxylase caused by predosing with vitamin D can be overcome with large amounts of the vitamin since increased circulating levels of 25-OH-D_3 are obviously observed as high doses of vitamin D are given (HADDAD and STAMP, 1974). The physiologic significance of this regulation remains unknown, although it is possible that vitamin D toxicity could be even greater were this regulation not in existence. The suggestion that there is a lack of regulation of 25-hydroxylation in the liver of birds (TUCKER et al., 1973) was later disproved since suppression could easily be demonstrated by merely increasing the dose of vitamin D to 20 units per chicken (BHATTACHARYYA and DELUCA, 1974a).

The circulating level of 25-OH-D_3 is a general reflection of the nutritional status of the organism with respect to vitamin D (PREECE et al., 1975; ARNAUD et al., 1976). Low levels of 25-OH-D_3 have been noted under conditions of inadequate vitamin D intake or production (PREECE et al., 1975; ARNAUD et al., 1976), intestinal malabsorption of vitamin D (PREECE et al., 1973), anticonvulsant therapy (STAMP et al., 1972) and steroid therapy (KLEIN et al., 1977). It is normal under conditions of renal osteodystrophy (BAYARD et al., 1973; OFFERMANN et al., 1974), X-linked hypophosphatemia (HADDAD et al., 1973a), and vitamin D-dependent rickets (FRASER et al., 1973).

II. Regulation of 1,25-Dihydroxyvitamin D_3 Production by Calcium and Parathyroid Hormone

There is no question that the most significant point of regulation of vitamin D metabolism is at the 1-hydroxylation stage. Regulation of this important step in vitamin D activation was first discovered by BOYLE et al. (1972b; 1973) shortly after the isolation and identification of 1,25-$(OH)_2D_3$ (HOLICK et al., 1971b). In this initial work BOYLE demonstrated that the in vivo conversion of 25-OH-D_3 to 1,25-$(OH)_2D_3$ was markedly and inversely dependent upon dietary calcium levels. Regulation of in vivo production of 1,25-$(OH)_2D_3$ was found only in the animals given small amounts of vitamin D_3. Vitamin D-deficient animals, on the other hand, showed high rates of conversion of 25-OH-D_3 to 1,25-$(OH)_2D_3$ except for those animals given 2 percent calcium plus lactose, in which case a suppression of 1,25-$(OH)_2D_3$ production could be observed in the 12 h test period. When 1-hydroxylation was suppressed by high dietary calcium, there was a corresponding increase in the appearance of another metabolite, which was later identified as 24,25-$(OH)_2D_3$ (HOLICK et al., 1972b). BOYLE and his colleagues readily surmised that the in vivo conversion of 25-OH-D_3 to the 1,25-$(OH)_2D_3$ was related to serum calcium concentration, independently of administration of vitamin D (Fig. 8). Thus the demand for calcium as registered by even slight hypocalcemia stimulated in vivo production of 1,25-$(OH)_2D_3$ and suppressed production of the 24,25-$(OH)_2D_3$. As animals became normal to hypercalcemic, 25-OH-D_3-1-hydroxylase was suppressed and 25-OH-D_3-24-hydroxylase, the presumed mechanism for inactivation, was stimulated (BOYLE et al., 1973). This basic discovery was soon confirmed by work in MacIntyre's laboratory, which highlighted the importance of vitamin D administration (GALANTE et al., 1972a; 1973). OMDAHL et al. (1972) then quickly demonstrated that the regulation of 1,25-$(OH)_2D_3$ accumulation in plasma and tissues in response to low dietary calcium was the direct result of increased activity of the 25-OH-D_3-1-hydroxylase as measured in vitro. OMDAHL and DELUCA (1971; 1972) then examined the question of strontium-induced rickets in which CORRADINO and WASSERMAN (1970) demonstrated a diminished intestinal calcium absorption and diminshed calcium-binding protein production. OMDAHL and DELUCA found that strontium brought about these suppressions by suppressing the 25-OH-D_3-1-hydroxylase, thereby shutting down production of 1,25-$(OH)_2D_3$ resulting in rachitogenesis, low calcium absorption, and low cal-

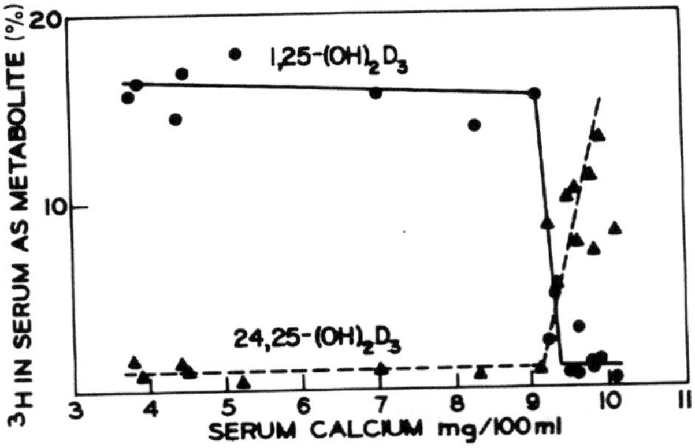

Fig. 8. The relationship between serum calcium concentration and the conversion of tritium-labeled 25-OH-D_3 to either 1,25-$(OH)_2D_3$ or 24,25-$(OH)_2D_3$. Rats were fed a variety of semipurified diets for a period of 2 weeks. At that time all animals were injected with tritium-labeled 25-OH-D_3, and 12 h later the plasma was removed, extracted, and chromatographed on Sephadex LH-20 to reveal ^{3}H-labeled 1,25-$(OH)_2D_3$ or 24,25-$(OH)_2D_3$. The amount of these metabolites in the plasma is plotted versus serum calcium concentration. Normal serum calcium concentration in these animals is 9.5 mg/100 ml

cium-binding protein production. The administration of 1,25-$(OH)_2D_3$ to strontium-dosed chickens overcame these inhibitions, clearly demonstrating the regulation of the 1-hydroxylase by strontium in the diet.

Garabedian et al. recognized that the relationship of serum calcium concentration to in vivo production of 1,25-$(OH)_2D_3$ might well be mediated by the parathyroid glands and parathyroid hormone secretion (Garabedian et al., 1972). In a series of experiments it was demonstrated that the hypocalcemic stimulation of 1,25-$(OH)_2D_3$ production could be eliminated by thyroparathyroidectomy and that 48 h following such surgery, the readministration of parathyroid hormone could result in recovery of 1,25-$(OH)_2D_3$ production to presurgical levels. They therefore demonstrated that the parathyroid hormone in some manner mediated the hypocalcemic stimulation of 1,25-$(OH)_2D_3$ production and the suppression of 24,25-$(OH)_2D_3$ accumulation (Garabedian et al., 1972). In support of these conclusions, Fraser and Kodicek (1973) demonstrated that the injection of parathyroid hormone caused a stimulation of the 25-OH-D_3-1-hydroxylase measured in vitro in the chick. Since these early experiments, confirmatory work on the effect of dietary calcium and of parathyroid hormone on the 25-OH-D_3-1-hydroxylase has been adequately provided (Henry et al., 1974; MacIntyre et al., 1975). In addition, high circulating levels of 1,25-$(OH)_2D_3$ in patients suffering from hyperparathyroidism and low levels in patients suffering from hypoparathyroidism and pseudohypoparathyroidism have been reported (Drezner et al., 1976; Haussler et al., 1976). There now is little doubt that 25-OH-D_3-1-hydroxylase is under the control of parathyroid hormone. Exactly how parathyroid hormone brings about its regulation remains largely unknown. Cyclic AMP administered to parathyroidectomized animals results in an increase in the 25-OH-D_3-1-hydroxylase just as if parathyroid hormone had been given (Suda et al., 1977). Furthermore, work carried out in thyroparathyroidectomized chickens given infusions of parathyroid hormone has shown that the hydroxylase is under direct control of this hormone (HORIUCHI et al., 1976; BOOTH et al., 1977). It seems reasonable to suspect that since the parathyroid hormone's action is mediated by cyclic AMP and cellular calcium in the kidney, the regulation of 25-OH-D_3-1-hydroxylase by parathyroid hormone involves a similar mechanism. However, confirmatory experiments for this conclusion are as yet lacking.

Because of the early work of BOYLE et al. (1971; 1972b) and of OMDAHL et al. (1972), it appeared that 25-OH-D_3-1-hydroxylase remains high in activity in the vitamin D-deficient state irrespective of dietary calcium and phosphorus. Thus regulation of this enzyme appeared to occur only after vitamin D administration. However, it has recently been demonstrated clearly by BOOTH and her colleagues (1977) and by SUDA and his colleagues that 25-OH-D_3-1-hydroxylase can be suppressed in vitamin D-deficient animals when they are parathyroidectomized and maintained with infusions of calcium (HORIUCHI et al., 1976). This suppressed level of 25-OH-D_3-1-hydroxylase can be restored by the readministration of parathyroid hormone. Of course, this point is of academic interest since in vitamin D deficiency there is no substrate upon which a hydroxylase can work; nevertheless, it represents an important point in our understanding of the regulatory mechanism. It is clear, however, that the production of 24,25-$(OH)_2D_3$ does not occur in the vitamin D-deficient animal (TANAKA and DELUCA, 1974). Thus it appears that some form of vitamin D must be present before this hydroxylase appears in appreciable amounts (TANAKA et al., 1975b). TANAKA et al. (1975b) provided evidence that 1,25-$(OH)_2D_3$ induces 25-OH-D_3-24-hydroxylase. A similar conclusion was reached by LARKINS et al. (1974a). An induction of such enzymatic activity in the kidney was supported by the observation of increased RNA synthesis in kidney tissue immediately following the administration of 1,25-$(OH)_2D_3$ (CHEN and DELUCA, 1973). α-Amanitin also prevents the 1,25-$(OH)_2D_3$-induced appearance of the 24-hydroxylase system, suggesting that a true induction is involved (LARKINS et al., 1975).

MACINTYRE and his colleagues have followed the apparent suppression of 25-OH-D_3-1-hydroxylase by 1,25-$(OH)_2D_3$ itself. There is no doubt that protein synthesis inhibitors and transcription inhibitors such as α-amanitin do prevent the 1,25-$(OH)_2D_3$-induced suppression of the 1-hydroxylase system (LARKINS et al., 1975). However, experiments by SUDA and his colleagues have demonstrated that constant infusions of parathyroid hormone prevent the suppression of 25-OH-D_3-1-hydroxylase by 1,25-$(OH)_2D_3$ (HORIUCHI et al., 1976). SUDA suggests that the suppression of 1-hydroxylase by 1,25-$(OH)_2D_3$ is mediated entirely by suppression of parathyroid hormone secretion. Although this may account in part for the suppression, SUDA and his colleagues have not explained why 1,25-$(OH)_2D_3$ will suppress 1-hydroxylase in hypophosphatemic animals where parathyroid hormone secretion is probably not a factor (TANAKA and DELUCA, 1974). It seems possible that although a good share of 1,25-$(OH)_2D_3$ suppression is mediated by suppression of parathyroid hormone secretion, it cannot account for the entire suppression phenomenon.

III. Regulation of 1,25-Dihydroxyvitamin D_3 Metabolism by Serum Phosphorus Concentration

Following the discovery that parathyroid hormone is involved in the hypocalcemic regulation of the 25-OH-D_3-1-hydroxylase, it was tempting to assume that the parathyroid hormone might serve as a trophic hormone for 1-hydroxylase. However, it became clear that animals maintained on low phosphorus diets had high levels of 25-OH-D_3-1-hydroxylase whether parathyroid glands were present or not (TANAKA and DELUCA, 1973). Furthermore, thyroparathyroidectomized animals who were then made hypophosphatemic either by dietary deprivation or by glucose loading had increased in vivo production of 1,25-$(OH)_2D_3$ even in the absence of parathyroid glands. There is no doubt, therefore, that there is increased accumulation of 1,25-$(OH)_2D_3$ in the plasma of animals on low phosphorus diets even in the absence of parathyroid glands. This result has been confirmed by direct analysis of plasma levels in rats and pigs (HUGHES et al., 1975; HAUSSLER et al., 1977). NORMAN and his colleagues (NORMAN et al., 1977) and HURWITZ and his colleagues (MONTECUCCOLI et al., 1977) have claimed that low phosphorus diets do not stimulate 25-OH-D_3-1-hydroxylase. Unfortunately, neither group used extremely low phosphorus diets, but certainly phosphate deprivation is much less effective in stimulating 1-hydroxylase than is the low calcium condition (BAXTER and DELUCA, 1976). Thus the degree of stimulation by phosphate deprivation is 3–5-fold whereas stimulation by low calcium diets is as much as 50-fold. There is obviously some additional factor involved in the accumulation of 1,25-$(OH)_2D_3$ under conditions of phosphate depletion. More recent results from our laboratory suggest that there is a decreased turnover of 1,25-$(OH)_2D_3$ and increased accumulation in both plasma and intestines of phosphate deprived animals (RIBOVICH and DELUCA, 1978b). Thus phosphate deprivation makes more effective the 1,25-$(OH)_2D_3$ that is produced. In any case, both hypocalcemia and hypophosphatemia stimulate mechanisms resulting in elevated plasma and tissue levels of 1,25-$(OH)_2D_3$, and subsequent increased plasma calcium and phosphate levels.

IV. Regulation of 25-Hydroxyvitamin D_3-24-Hydroxylase by 1,25-Dihydroxyvitamin D_3, Parathyroid Hormone, and Ambient Calcium Concentration

As pointed out in the previous section, it seems clear that 1,25-$(OH)_2D_3$ has a direct role in inducing renal 25-OH-D_3-24-hydroxylase and may also have a direct effect on the suppression of 25-OH-D_3-1-hydroxylase. The mechanisms of these regulations remain largely unknown. A study of the regulation of 25-OH-D_3-hydroxylases has demonstrated its marked suppression by the presence of the parathyroid hormone (TANAKA et al., 1975b; JUAN and DELUCA, 1977) and by means of high calcium diets (BOYLE et al., 1971). This is counteracted by the inducing effect of 1,25-$(OH)_2D_3$ (JUAN and DELUCA, 1977; TANAKA et al., 1975b). It has been possible to culture monkey kidney cells which in turn produce 24,25-$(OH)_2D_3$ in vitro (JUAN and DELUCA, 1977). The production of 24,25-$(OH)_2D_3$ is stimulated by 1,25-$(OH)_2D_3$ and by increased ambient calcium concentration in the culture fluid. Furthermore, it is markedly suppressed by small amounts of parathyroid hormone. These tissue culture results again confirm the independent effects of these three agents in regulating 24-hydroxylase. However, they do not provide insight regarding the mechanism nor do they necessarily extend in a reciprocal manner to 1-hydroxylase. There is a need for a tissue culture system that is clearly able to produce on a long-term basis 1,25-$(OH)_2D_3$ and that is sensitive to the in vivo regulators. This is under development in a number of laboratories, which should hopefully confirm some of the in vivo data. Undoubtedly, however, the tissue culture systems will not provide the molecular mechanisms of regulation; these will require much more sophisticated molecular biology and enzymology.

V. Regulation of Vitamin D Metabolism by the Sex Hormones

One of the most dramatic changes in calcium metabolism can be found in the egg-laying birds (BELL and FREEMAN, 1971). It is well known that birds during the egg production phase of their lives will transfer as much as 1 g of calcium to the egg shell in the course of 1 or 2 h. The source of this calcium is generally medullary bone with some dietary calcium. The remarkable shifts in calcium during this cycle undoubtedly produce profound changes in the endocrine systems involved in regulating calcium metabolism. Initially KENNY et al. (1974) suggested that the 25-OH-D_3-1-hydroxylase might be elevated in birds when the egg was found in a particular position in the oviduct. This led to an investigation of the changes in the renal 25-OH-D_3-1-hydroxylase during the egg production phase of the avian species (TANAKA et al., 1976b; CASTILLO et al., 1977; BAKSI and KENNY, 1977). Using the Japanese quail, it could be demonstrated that egg-laying females had high levels of 25-OH-D_3-1-hydroxylase whereas males of the same age, the same group, and under the same conditions had low levels of 1-hydroxylase and significant levels of the 25-OH-D_3-24-hydroxylase. If an injection of estradiol was given to mature male quails, within 24 h there was a high level of 25-OH-D_3-1-hydroxylase and a suppression of 24-hydroxylase. Because this response was not found in immature male quails, injections of both testosterone and estradiol were given. Treatment with a combination of these two hormones resulted in a marked stimulation of 1-hydroxylase. A detailed investigation of this phenomenon in castrated male birds led to the unequivocal demonstration that the estradiol stimulation of the 1-hydroxylase system required the presence of testosterone. Testosterone could be replaced by progesterone and the presence of all three hormones produced maximal responses in the 25-OH-D_3-1-hydroxylase (CASTILLO et al., unpublished).

The response to estradiol is highly specific, not being produced by any other hormone. In examining the egg-laying cycle, it became clear, however, that the formation of the medullary bone in maturing female birds is not related to 25-OH-D_3-1-hydroxylase or plasma levels of 1,25-$(OH)_2D_3$, but rather to the presence of estradiol and testosterone (TANAKA et al., unpublished results). It was only when egg production began, with the consequent resorption of medullary bone, that the renal 25-OHD$_3$-1-hydroxylase was markedly elevated. It seems likely that the increased 25-OH-D$_3$-1-hydroxylase activity results in improved intestinal absorption of calcium and also facilitates resorption of medullary bone, providing calcium for egg production. After the egg shell has been completed, medullary bone is depleted. During the next several hours formation of medullary bone is followed by suppression of plasma 1,25-(OH)$_2$D$_3$ levels. When the next egg is formed, 25-OH-D$_3$-1-hydroxylase is stimulated once again. It seems likely that the cyclic production of 1,25-(OH)$_2$D$_3$ plays an important role in intestinal calcium absorption and in medullary bone resorption in egg-laying birds. Thus it might be expected that under conditions where there is an excessive demand on calcium metabolism, other endocrine systems may in some direct or indirect manner stimulate 25-OH-D$_3$-1-hydroxylase thereby providing more 1,25-(OH)$_2$D$_3$ to increase intestinal utilization of calcium and possibly to increase the utilization of calcium from the bone fluid compartment. It seems likely that one can suspect increased circulating levels of 1,25-(OH)$_2$D$_3$ during rapid phases of growth (TANAKA et al., unpublished results), and during pregnancy and lactation. It seems possible that these conditions might also directly or indirectly affect calcium metabolism. In fact, SPANOS and MACINTYRE (1977) reported prolactin injections stimulate 25-OH-D$_3$-1-hydroxylase in chickens, and diabetes in rats has been shown to be related to low circulating levels of 1,25-(OH)$_2$D$_3$, giving low rates of intestinal calcium absorption (SCHNEIDER et al., 1976; 1977). There is indeed much more to be expected in this area of endocrine interrelationships that impinge upon the vitamin D endocrine system for generation or mobilization of increased amounts of calcium needed for specialized functions.

VI. Mechanisms of Regulation of the Renal Hydroxylases

There has been a great deal of interest generated in the molecular mechanisms whereby the vitamin D hydroxylases of the kidney are regulated by the parathyroid hormone, by phosphate deprivation, by the sex hormones, and by 1,25-(HD)$_2$D$_3$ itself (DELUCA, 1975). A number of attempts have been made to draw conclusions based on the addition of calcium ions and phosphate ions to kidney mitochondria incubation in vitro. Other experiments have involved isolated renal tubules (BIKLE et al., 1975; BIKLE and RASMUSSEN, 1975; COLSTON et al., 1973; LARKINS et al., 1974b; SUDA et al., 1973; HENRY and NORMAN, 1976). Again, manipulations of ion concentrations and hormone additions have been evaluated. These experiments have been highly controversial and contradictory. It is impossible to sort out exactly what is the physiologically meaningful experiment, if any. Perhaps the most telling argument is that no minute-to-minute regulation of the hydroxylases has been demonstrated in vivo. In fact, it seems clear that, in view of the relatively long lifetime of 1,25-(OH)$_2$D$_3$, short term regulation is unlikely to be physiologically significant. Of the in vivo regulations, it is clear that the most important are those which require many hours to elicit. Thus short-term experiments with calcium additions to mitochondria, phosphate additions to mitochondria, parathyroid hormone additions, etc., are not likely to have any physiologic meaning—if they can be reproduced at all. For this reason, this author will not review the massive amount of data that has been published in this area. It is also known that the lifetimes of both 1-hydroxylase and 24-hydroxylase can be measured in a matter of hours (TANAKA et al., 1972; TSAI et al., 1973). It is therefore probable that the two hydroxylase systems turn over rapidly and that the regulation may well be on the synthesis and degradation of the enzymes. On the other hand, it is possible that a regulator substance is either synthesized or degraded under the influence of the parathyroid hormone, calcium, cyclic AMP, and other factors. Furthermore it is not known whether the sex hormones act directly on the hydroxylases or whether their actions are mediated by the parathyroid glands (TANAKA et al., 1976b; CASTILLO et al., 1977; BAKSI and KENNY, 1977). Similarly the influence of diabetes on 1-hydroxylase may be indirect, affecting some of the other known regulators of vitamin D metabolism. During the next decade much work can be expected in the area of regulation of the vitamin D hydroxylases, both descriptive and mechanistic. However, progress will probably be slow since much work has been expended on the role of ACTH in steroidogenesis without that system being fully elucidated. Undoubtedly detailed enzymology of the hydroxylases must be accomplished before mechanisms can be examined regarding the hydroxylases of the kidney in a serious manner.

VII. Calcium Homeostatic Mechanisms Involving the Vitamin D Endocrine System

(Fig. 9)

With the discovery of the vitamin D endocrine system of the kidney has come a renewed possibility that a detailed understanding of the calcium homeostatic system can be achieved. Certainly, one must now include the vitamin D endocrine system centrally in the calcium homeostatic mechanism, not only because vitamin D is intimately involved with the parathyroid hormone in maintaining plasma calcium concentration, but also because it is intimately involved in the regulation of intestinal calcium absorption, which provides the only means that the organism has to conserve its skeleton by sequestering environmental calcium.

Before this mechanism can be discussed, it is important to realize that a third hormone not yet discussed is also of importance. That hormone, calcitonin, is perhaps the most recently discovered of the calcium homeostatic hormones. Its function is believed to be primarily at the bone site, where it suppresses the mobilization of calcium and phosphate from bone (TAYLOR, 1970). The mechanism whereby this is brought about remains largely unknown. This hormone is secreted in response to hypercalcemia and in response to gastrointestinal hormones (HIRSCH et al., 1975). In fact, its chief function is believed to relate to postprandial hypercalcemia in which the gastrointestinal hormone causes secretion of calcitonin which then suppresses calcium coming from bone, permitting maximum utilization of dietary calcium and maximum deposit of dietary calcium in bone (DEFTOS, 1978). It had been postulated that calcitonin might influence vitamin D metabolism. Experiments were carried out by GALANTE et al. (1972b) in which large amounts of calcitonin appeared to increase produc-

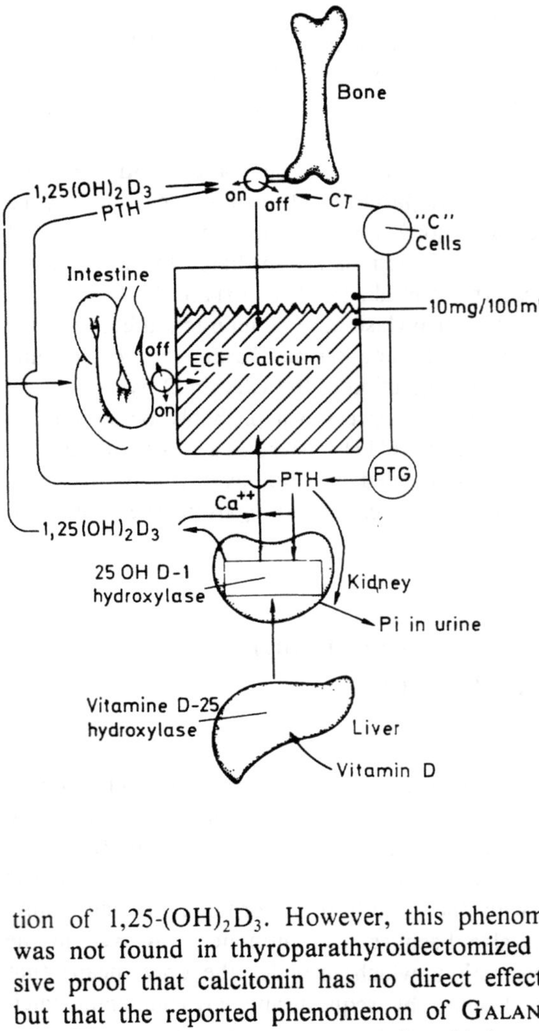

Fig. 9. A diagrammatic representation of the calcium homeostatic mechanisms involving the vitamin D endocrine system. Note that hypocalcemia stimulates parathyroid hormone secretion, which in turn stimulates the kidney to produce 1,25-$(OH)_2$-D_3. 1,25-$(OH)_2D_3$ stimulates intestinal calcium absorption and together with the parathyroid hormone stimulates the mobilization of calcium from the bone fluid compartment and the reabsorption of calcium in the renal tubules

tion of 1,25-$(OH)_2D_3$. However, this phenomenon, which could be reproduced, was not found in thyroparathyroidectomized animals, and there is now conclusive proof that calcitonin has no direct effect on renal 25-OH-D_3-1-hydroxylase but that the reported phenomenon of GALANTE et al. was the result of a countersecretion of endogenous parathyroid hormone reacting to the hypocalcemia brought about by the injection of large amounts of calcitonin (LORENC et al., 1977).

Another important major factor of interest is the ability of the intestine to adapt to dietary calcium (NICOLAYSEN, 1943; NICOLAYSEN et al., 1953). With the discovery of the regulation of 1,25-$(OH)_2D_3$ production by dietary calcium, came the concept that the endogenous factor, which NICOLAYSEN postulated to direct intestinal calcium absorption, might be increased production of 1,25-$(OH)_2D_3$ (NICOLAYSEN et al., 1953). Thus in response to low dietary calcium or great needs for calcium in calcification of bone, slight hypocalcemia would bring about increased parathyroid hormone secretion that in turn would stimulate production of 1,25-$(OH)_2D_3$ (BOYLE et al., 1972b). 1,25-$(OH)_2D_3$ would then stimulate intestinal calcium absorption. In support of this concept it has been demonstrated that the administration of 1,25-$(OH)_2D_3$ eliminates the ability of animals to adjust their intestinal calcium absorption in relationship to dietary calcium levels (RIBOVICH and DELUCA,

1975). Furthermore, parathyroidectomy with the subsequent administration of an exogenous but constant source of parathyroid hormone also eliminates the ability of the intestine to adapt to dietary calcium levels (RIBOVICH and DELUCA, 1976). Thus the endogenous factor of NICOLAYSEN is almost certain to be the parathyroid gland system plus the vitamin D endocrine system.

Following the demonstration that the parathyroid hormone is responsible for stimulating 1,25-$(OH)_2D_3$ production in response to hypocalcemia, the question arose as to whether almost all of the effects of the parathyroid hormone could be accounted for by its stimulation of the production of 1,25-$(OH)_2D_3$ (GARABEDIAN et al., 1974). To test this possibility the response of intestine and bone to 1,25-$(OH)_2D_3$ was tested in the presence and absence of parathyroid hormone (GARABEDIAN et al., 1974). It was demonstrated that intestinal calcium absorption responds only to 1,25-$(OH)_2D_3$, and does not respond to parathyroid hormone either in the presence or absence of 1,25-$(OH)_2D_3$. Thus the stimulation of intestinal calcium absorption by the parathyroid hormone is mediated by the production of 1,25-$(OH)_2D_3$. On the other hand, the mobilization of calcium from bone requires both parathyroid hormone and 1,25-$(OH)_2D_3$. Similarly, the reabsorption of calcium in the renal tubule appears to involve both 1,25-$(OH)_2D_3$ (SUTTON et al., 1977) and the parathyroid hormone (KLEEMAN et al., 1961).

If one then assembles these facts into a diagram of the calcium homeostatic mechanism as shown in Fig. 9, the following points can be made. Under conditions of hypocalcemia, the parathyroid glands secrete parathyroid hormone which in turn specifically binds to kidney, liver, and bone (ZULL and REPKE, 1972; NEUMAN et al., 1975). Significantly, no labeled parathyroid hormone is bound specifically in the intestine. In the kidney the parathyroid hormone stimulates renal reabsorption of calcium (KLEEMAN et al., 1961) and causes a phosphate diuresis (FORTE et al., 1976). In addition, it stimulates 1,25-$(OH)_2D_3$ production. The 1,25-$(OH)_2D_3$ stimulates intestinal calcium absorption and together with the secreted parathyroid hormone stimulates the transfer of calcium from the bone fluid compartment to the extracellular fluid compartment. These three sources of calcium cause an elevation of plasma calcium concentration, suppressing parathyroid hormone secretion, thereby shutting down the entire calcium mobilizing system. On the other hand, if hypercalcemia is found or results, there is a secretion of calcitonin from the C cells of the thyroid which then suppresses mobilization of calcium from bone and probably stimulates excretion of calcium and phosphorus in the kidney (MAIER, 1974). These factors bring down the plasma calcium and phosphorus concentrations to the normal range.

There are two important facets of the calcium homeostatic mechanism that should be mentioned. Undoubtedly there are both short-term and long-term regulatory phenomena involved in the increased utilization of calcium from the intestine. It is known that the vitamin D endocrine system requires many hours before it reacts to stimulation by parathyroid hormone (GARABEDIAN et al., 1972). Furthermore, the action of 1,25-$(OH)_2D_3$ requires hours and its lifetime can be measured in hours if not days. It is obvious that this system does not react sufficiently to quickly adjust changes in serum calcium concentration. There must, therefore, be a more rapidly acting mechanism. The secretion of parathyroid hormone occurs within minutes in response to hypocalcemic stimuli and the lifetime action of this hormone can be measured in minutes (ZULL and REPKE, 1972; NEUMAN et al., 1975). Thus perturbations in serum calcium are adjusted quickly by appropriate secretions of parathyroid hormone that would improve renal reabsorption of calcium in the presence of the existent $1,25\text{-}(OH)_2D_3$. Similarly the mobilization of calcium from the bone fluid compartment can also be stimulated by parathyroid hormone acting in concert with existent $1,25\text{-}(OH)_2D_3$ to correct the hypocalcemia. If there is continued stimulation of the renal system with parathyroid hormone, increased amounts of $1,25\text{-}(OH)_2D_3$ must ultimately result. This long-term-acting hormone now throws into play the one organ that can bring calcium into this system from the environment, namely, the intestine. In addition, increased levels of $1,25\text{-}(OH)_2D_3$ in the kidney and in bone must increase the sensitivity of these organs to the secreted parathyroid hormone. Thus under conditions of more chronic stimulation, the $1,25\text{-}(OH)_2D_3$ system provides the mechanism whereby environmental calcium can be made available, thus protecting the skeleton from continued loss of calcium. In the absence of this mechanism it is obvious that the parathyroid system will continually raid the calcium in the skeleton, and if this continues, bone mass will decrease, causing osteopenia, thus perhaps contributing to osteoporosis.

F. Functions of Vitamin D

I. Intestine

1. Calcium Transport

From the early work of NICOLAYSEN it was firmly established that vitamin D improves intestinal calcium absorption (NICOLAYSEN, 1937a, b, c; NICOLAYSEN et al., 1953). NICOLAYSEN and his associates further demonstrated conclusively that vitamin D is essential for the ability of the intestine to adapt its intestinal calcium absorption to the needs for calcium (NICOLAYSEN et al., 1953). These two fundamental biological observations still remain today to be elucidated in molecular detail. Following the work of NICOLAYSEN, several investigators using a variety of techniques confirmed the idea that vitamin D increases intestinal calcium absorption (WASSERMAN, 1963). However, little progress was made until SCHACHTER and ROSEN introduced the technique of everted intestinal sacs in vitro as a technique to measure calcium transport (SCHACHTER and ROSEN, 1959). Using this technique, these pioneering investigations revealed that vitamin D increases the transport of calcium against a concentration gradient in a process which required metabolic energy and thus appeared to be active transport (DOWDLE et al., 1960; SCHACHTER, 1963). SCHACHTER and colleagues continued their investigations and demonstrated that the ability of the small intestine to transport calcium was not only dependent upon vitamin D, but was also modulated by dietary calcium levels in support of the early conclusions of NICOLAYSEN (KIMBERG et al., 1961). HARRISON and HARRISON (1965) confirmed the everted intestinal sac work of SCHACHTER and his colleagues but introduced the concept that vitamin D might not function at the active transport site but might rather increase the permeability of small intestine to calcium. This controversy has not yet been resolved, and the possibility remains that vitamin D may change the permeability of intestinal membrane to calcium and that the active transport mechanism might be vitamin D independent. Still other in vitro experiments have firmly established that calcium is transported against an electrochemical potential gradient and is a saturable process by the criteria of USSING (SCHACHTER, 1963; WASSERMAN et al., 1961; ADAMS and NORMAN, 1970; MARTIN and DELUCA, 1969a). Although the duodenum appears to be the most active site of intestinal calcium transport in response to vitamin D, it appears that vitamin D stimulates the transport of calcium throughout the small and to some extent large intestine (HARRISON and HARRISON, 1969). The calcium transport process requires sodium ions, at least as measured in vitro by the everted sac technique (MARTIN and DELUCA, 1969b; HARRISON and HARRISON, 1963). In the absence of sodium ions, calcium accumulates in intestinal tissue and is not expelled into the serosal medium. Although these results suggest that sodium is required for the expulsion of calcium across the basal-lateral membrane of the intestinal villus cells, the possibility that failure to expel sodium is the result of muscle accumulation has not been adequately excluded (N. KENDRICK, personal communication). In any case, it seems clear that sodium is required to observe active calcium transport in the small intestine in response to vitamin D.

The site of vitamin D function in the intestinal epithelial cells has received some attention. In early work SCHACHTER's group came to the conclusion that vitamin D increases the transport of calcium both at the brush border surface and at the basal-lateral membrane (SCHACHTER et al., 1966). On the other hand, other investigators have not found evidence for a vitamin D-dependent transport across the basal-lateral membrane (MARTIN and DELUCA, 1969a, b; WALLING and ROTHMAN, 1969; 1973). The possibility, therefore, remains open as to whether vitamin D has a function at the basal-lateral membrane. Almost all evidence is consistent with the idea that vitamin D in some way affects the initial transfer of calcium across the brush border surface. SAMPSON et al. (1970) reported that vitamin D-deficient intestine shows granules of what is believed to be calcium at the brush border surface of the small intestine and that following vitamin D administration, these granules disappear and, instead, granules appear in intestinal epithelial mitochondria. The experiments of MARTIN and DELUCA (1969a), WALLING and ROTHMAN (1969; 1973), and NORMAN and co-workers (ADAMS and NORMAN, 1970; ADAMS et al., 1970) are also consistent with the idea that an early event in the uptake of calcium by the intestinal epithelium is affected by vitamin D administration. In an interesting series of experiments, ADAMS et al. (1970), using the antibiotic filipin, were able to render the small intestine of vitamin D-deficient chicks similar to the intestine of vitamin D-supplemented chicks, suggesting that the brush border membrane is the chief barrier in calcium transport in the vitamin D-deficient state. To summarize, therefore, there appears to be uniform agreement that vitamin D affects some process near or at the brush border membrane surface to facilitate the transport of calcium.

Over the past ten years, several attempts have been made to identify the substance that is responsible for the vitamin D-mediated increase in calcium transport at the brush border surface. The most notable of these efforts has been that of WASSERMAN and his colleagues who discovered in 1966 the existence of a calcium-binding protein in the intestines of chicks given vitamin D (WASSERMAN and TAYLOR, 1966). In the absence of vitamin D this protein is absent and appears following vitamin D administration. This protein has been isolated in pure form and in the case of the chick it has a molecular weight of 24,000 (WASSERMAN et al., 1974), and its amino acid composition is known, revealing a high concentration of dicarboxylic amino acids, namely, aspartate, which probably accounts for its calcium-binding activity (WASSERMAN et al., 1974; WASSERMAN and FEHER, 1977). It has no phosphate, and the chick protein binds four calcium ions per mole of protein (WASSERMAN and FEHER, 1977). The calcium is bound to two high-affinity sites and two low-affinity sites. The mammalian counterpart of the calcium-binding protein has also been isolated from the rat (DRESCHER and DELUCA, 1971a; BRUNS et al., 1977), from the pig (ARNOLD et al., 1977), and from the bovine (FULLMER and WASSERMAN, 1973). The rat protein has a molecular weight of 8,000–12,000. A great deal of work has been done on all of these proteins and much is known concerning them. A major question is, however, whether this protein does in fact represent the carrier protein for calcium which is made in response to vitamin D. WASSERMAN and his colleagues put forth the powerful argument in that in the chick at least the calcium-binding protein is absent in the deficient state and appears following vitamin D administration (MORRISSEY and

Wasserman, 1971; Ingersoll and Wasserman, 1971; Corradino et al., 1971a, b). The level of calcium-binding protein correlates with the level of intestinal calcium transport as affected by strontium, dietary calcium, and other factors that affect intestinal calcium absorption. On the other hand, calcium-binding protein is not absent in rats in the vitamin D-deficient state (Bruns et al., 1977; Drescher and DeLuca, 1971a). Furthermore, large amounts of vitamin D are needed to elevate the calcium-binding protein of rat small intestine to significant degrees (Drescher and DeLuca, 1971a). Perhaps the most powerful argument against the calcium-binding protein carrier concept for vitamin D function is the observation that the appearance of calcium-binding protein in the small intestine does not correlate with the appearance of intestinal calcium transport. This was originally discovered by Harmeyer and DeLuca (1969) and has recently been reaffirmed by Spencer et al. (1976). In fact, if one studies the appearance of intestinal calcium-binding protein in response to a single dose of 1,25-$(OH)_2D_3$ to chicks and using a very sensitive antibody to detect calcium-binding protein, it is clear that calcium-binding protein is not detected at the time intestinal calcium transport is initiated. Furthermore, following decay of intestinal calcium transport in these chicks, the calcium-binding protein remains at a high level while calcium transport returns to predosing levels. Originally Ebel et al. (1969) countered the argument of Harmeyer and DeLuca by stating that the Chelex method for determining calcium-binding protein was not sensitive enough to permit detection of small amounts of calcium-binding protein. With their antibody to calcium-binding protein, a correlation could be found between the initial calcium transport response and the appearance of calcium-binding protein. This, however, appears not to be borne out by the work of Lawson and his colleagues (1969). Besides this problem it is known that glucocorticoids increase the calcium-binding protein level in small intestine whereas they diminish the calcium transport activity (Kimberg et al., 1971). Finally, the work of Drescher and DeLuca (1971b) and more recently of Bruns and Avioli (1975) in the rat has shown that incorporation of amino acids into the calcium-binding protein in the rat does not correlate with the de novo synthesis of a calcium transport substance required for vitamin D-induced calcium transport. It is, therefore, not clear whether the calcium-binding protein which was discovered by Wasserman does in fact carry out the role of vitamin D in the transfer of calcium across the brush border membrane. Another problem with the calcium-binding protein has been the exact cellular location of the protein. Initially, Taylor and Wasserman, concludes that using immunofluorescence microscopy the calcium-binding protein was in the goblet cells of intestine and along the surface of the microvilli (Taylor and Wasserman, 1970). Other results from Morrissey and his group conflict with this concept (Morrissey et al., 1975). In their studies, calcium-binding protein was found widely distributed, including in the cytosol of the intestinal villus cells. Another problem with the calcium-binding protein is that it is found in other tissues including brain (Taylor, 1974a), and in the case of brain, the amount of calcium-binding protein does not appear to be under the influence of vitamin D. If vitamin D is a hormonal substance that leads to the transcription of the gene coding for the calcium-binding protein, it is difficult to understand how some tissues in the absence of vitamin D would have sufficient amounts of this calcium-binding protein.

Because of the questions surrounding the calcium-binding protein, other attempts at understanding the vitamin D-induced calcium transport have been made. Perhaps of historical interest has been the problem of intestinal alkaline phosphatase, which is primarily located in the brush border membranes. There is no doubt that alkaline phosphatase is present in the vitamin D-deficient state (PILEGGI et al., 1955). The level of intestinal alkaline phosphatase is increased by vitamin D, but its appearance does not correlate well with intestinal calcium transport (EBEL et al., 1969; WASSERMAN and TAYLOR, 1972). Recent work indicates that the vitamin D metabolite, $1,25\text{-}(OH)_2D_3$, might influence the isoenzyme proportions in the microvillus of small intestine. Thus MORIUCHI and DELUCA (1976) first demonstrated that in the absence of vitamin D a 220,000 molecular weight protein was found containing alkaline phosphatase activity. Following $1,25\text{-}(OH)_2D_3$ administration this protein band disappeared from disc gel patterns and instead a protein with slower migration and containing alkaline phosphatase activity appeared in the profiles. In addition, the butanol extracts of intestinal brush borders contained both alkaline phosphatase and calcium-binding activities. Recently MORIUCHI et al. (1977) showed that the addition of sialic acid to the alkaline phosphatase of brush borders is responsible for the change in electrophoretic mobility. This process is activated by calcium. Thus it appears that this change is secondary to calcium transport.

SCHACHTER and his colleagues (1966) studied a calcium-binding protein complex that appears following vitamin D administration and that may play a role in calcium transport. Another approach has been the use of double label techniques. DRESCHER and DELUCA (1971b) reasoned that one could follow the appearance of radio-labeled proteins in response to vitamin D using the double label technique of FOX and KENNEDY. Unfortunately, after injection of amino acids in vivo, no new protein containing a large amount of labeled amino acids following vitamin D administration could be detected. However, recently this technique has been more sophisticatedly applied by LAWSON and his colleagues using in vitro incubation with the labeled amino acids (WILSON and LAWSON, 1977).

With this technique they have detected a 44,000 molecular weight protein that becomes labeled in response to $1,25\text{-}(OH)_2D_3$ at about the time one would expect a calcium transfer protein to appear. This protein disappears and an 88,000 molecular weight protein makes its appearance in the brush border. The 88,000 molecular weight protein correlates very well with intestinal calcium transport while the 44,000 molecular weight protein appears prior to the calcium transport response. Whether either of these proteins plays a role in calcium transport remains to be determined. In any case it is clear that the carrier responsible for the calcium transport process in response to vitamin D remains to be elucidated. With the availability of the active form of vitamin D and with modern techniques of immunology and biochemistry, in the next decade the carrier responsible for vitamin D function should be identified.

Some attempts have been made to demonstrate that vitamin D plays a role in lipid metabolism and composition of the brush border membranes. Early work with ^{32}P revealed that vitamin D influenced the incorporation of ^{32}P into certain phospholipid fractions (THOMPSON and DELUCA, 1964). This phenomenon appeared to be secondary to changes in inorganic phosphorus transfer. More recently, however, GOODMAN et al. put forth two concepts: One is that the cholesterol esters are altered by vitamin D administration (GOODMAN et al., 1972) and, more recently, the idea that certain phospholipids might be altered by $1,25\text{-}(OH)_2D_3$ administration (RASMUSSEN et al., 1977). Whether these are primary or secondary and whether they play a role in calcium transport again remains unknown.

2. Factors which Regulate Intestinal Calcium Transport by Regulating Vitamin D Conversion to 1,25-$(OH)_2D_3$

As discussed previously, the most important of these factors is dietary calcium and plasma calcium concentration. The need for calcium in some manner stimulates the efficiency of intestinal calcium transport. It appears certain that a major if not entire portion of this phenomenon can be accounted for by the slight hypocalcemia stimulating the parathyroid glands and the parathyroid hormone stimulating the production of 1,25-$(OH)_2D_3$. 1,25-$(OH)_2D_3$ then stimulates intestinal calcium absorption. In a reverse manner, high calcium diets bring about a suppression of parathyroid hormone secretion, a suppression of 1,25-$(OH)_2D_3$ production, and thus suppression of intestinal calcium absorption. This concept of the NICOLAYSEN endogenous factor was put forth by BOYLE in 1971 and has been confirmed by the following experiments. BAR and WASSERMAN, using dihydrotachysterol as an analog of 1,25-$(OH)_2D_3$, demonstrated that chicks were unable to elicit the adaptation of intestinal calcium absorption to dietary calcium when given this form of vitamin D (BAR and WASSERMAN, 1973). Similarly, OMDAHL and DELUCA (1977) with the chick and RIBOVICH and DELUCA (1975) with the rat demonstrated that exogenous sources of 1,25-$(OH)_2D_3$ eliminate the ability of these animals to increase their intestinal calcium absorption in response to low dietary calcium.

There has been considerable controversy surrounding the idea that the parathyroid glands are involved in the ability of the intestine to adapt to dietary calcium. Some investigators of considerable reputation have reported that parathyroidectomized rats possess the ability to adapt their calcium absorption to dietary calcium (FAVUS et al., 1974). On the other hand, other investigators are unable to confirm this result. In fact, WINTER et al. (1972) and SHAH and DRAPER (1966) demonstrated that the parathyroid glands are involved. However, PENTO and KENNY (1970) found that during the week following parathyroidectomy, the animals were unable to adapt but after a week, adaptation occurred. Unfortunately the problem with parathyroidectomy is the uncertainty of removal of all of the parathyroid tissue. In the author's experience, complete removal of the parathyroid tissue renders animals incapable of surviving the insult of low dietary calcium. It would appear that the survivors under such circumstances have sufficient amounts of parathyroid tissue to permit their survival. Thus the experiments of FAVUS et al. are subject to the criticism that only the survivors of thyroparathyroidectomy were studied. To circumvent this problem, RIBOVICH and DELUCA (1976) not only thyroparathyroidectomized the animals but replaced the thyroid hormone and provided a constant exogenous amount of parathyroid hormone. In these animals no adaptation to dietary calcium could be observed. Furthermore, one could easily demonstrate that the maintenance of calcium adaptation to low dietary calcium could be eliminated by parathyroidectomy and the initial event in adaptation could also be eliminated by thyroparathyroidectomy. It therefore appears virtually certain that the parathyroid glands play an important role in the ability of the intestine to adapt its efficiency of absorption to the level of dietary calcium or to the needs for calcium.

As pointed out previously, dietary strontium is known to induce a strontium rickets, which is associated with reduced intestinal calcium absorption and reduced calcium-binding protein. It is now clear that the feeding of strontium inhibits 25-OH-D_3-1-hydroxylase or rather suppresses its activity, resulting in low levels of 1,25-$(OH)_2D_3$ giving low intestinal calcium absorption and diminished levels of calcium-binding protein (OMDAHL et al., 1972; OMDAHL and DELUCA, 1972). This can be overcome by the administration of 1,25-$(OH)_2D_3$. Furthermore, in vitro and in vivo data have been provided which show that the strontium-fed animals do have suppressed 25-OH-D_3-1-hydroxylase and elevated 25-OH-D_3-24-hydroxylase levels.

Cattle and horses that were fed the plants *Solanum glaucophyllum* and *Cestrum diurnum* developed vitamin D toxicity (WASSERMAN, 1975). These substances were studied for many years and, following the discovery of 1,25-$(OH)_2D_3$, it appeared that *Solanum glaucophyllum* and *Cestrum diurnum* material in many way acted similarly to 1,25-$(OH)_2D_3$. It was, therefore, demonstrated that these substances are active in anephric, vitamin D-deficient animals in stimulating intestinal calcium absorption; additonally, they are active in overcoming strontium inhibition of intestinal calcium absorption (WASSERMAN, 1974), and, in general, elicit vitamin D toxicity symptoms. Using a radioreceptor method for determination of 1,25-$(OH)_2D_3$ in tissue, PETERLIK and WASSERMAN (1975) and NAPOLI et al. (1977a) were able to demonstrate that the feeding of *Solanum glaucophyllum* to animals resulted in marked elevations in plasma and intestinal levels of 1,25-$(OH)_2D_3$, revealing that the *Solanum glaucophyllum* contributed some form of vitamin D resulting in high amounts of 1,25-$(OH)_2D_3$ in vitamin D-deficient animals. Since the animals were deficient in vitamin D one could exclude factors that might stimulate conversion of the vitamin D to its active form. Furthermore, the fact that the *Solanum glaucophyllum* extracts were active in anephric animals and in strontium-fed chicks gave confidence that the compound was either 1α-OH-D_3 or 1,25-$(OH)_2D_3$ in a conjugated form to permit water solubility. WASSERMAN and his colleagues were then able to hydrolyze sufficient amounts of the *Solanum glaucophyllum* material and to obtain a purified sample of 1,25-$(OH)_2D_3$, and its presence could then be confirmed by mass spectrometry (WASSERMAN et al., 1976). Exactly how 1,25-$(OH)_2D_3$ is conjugated and to what remains unknown. Similar results have been published for *Cestrum diurnum* (HUGHES et al., 1977). Thus this agent acts to increase intestinal calcium absorption by providing a water-soluble form of 1,25-$(OH)_2D_3$ or a 1-hydroxylated precursor.

Scientists at the Procter and Gamble Company have developed a series of compounds known as diphosphonates. These compounds have a phosphorus–carbon–phosphorus bond which causes them to resemble pyrophosphate. These substances bind to hydroxyapatite, and it had been believed that these materials could coat the mineral component of bone, thereby inhibiting bone resorption or inhibiting further bone crystal formation (FLEISCH et al., 1968). It has been used therapeutically in the treatment of such diseases as osteitis osificans and more recently Paget's disease (CANFIELD et al., 1977). When given in large amounts, ethane-1-hydroxy-1,1-diphosphonate (EHDP) produces a rachitic-like condition in young animals (BONJOUR et al., 1972) or an osteomalacic condition in adult animals. At these doses the diphosphonate inhibits intestinal calcium absorption, and this inhibition can be overcome by the administration of 1,25-$(OH)_2D_3$ (BONJOUR et al., 1973; 1975; 1976; BAXTER et al., 1974). Subsequent experiments have demonstrated that EHDP inhibits 25-OH-D_3-1-hydroxylase, probably in a systemic fashion (BAXTER et al., 1974). Thus doses of as low as 10 mg/kg injected subcutaneously will, after one week, cause very marked inhibition of this hydroxylase. Doses as low as 4 mg/kg might, on prolonged administration, also give suppressed 25-OH-D_3-1-hydroxylase. However, these levels are far in excess of those used in the treatment of Paget's disease. In addition, recent results have shown that plasma levels of 1,25-$(OH)_2D_3$ are not suppressed (DELUCA et al., unpublished) in Paget's disease patients by doses of 10–20 mg of EHDP per kg body weight given orally (CANFIELD et al., 1977). However, it should be recognized that only 3 percent of the dose is absorbed from the oral route (KING et al., 1971). In any case, it appears that diphosphonates at very high levels will indirectly suppress 25-OH-D_3-1-hydroxylase. The mechanism of this suppression remains largely unknown.

There has been some attention regarding the glucocorticoid inhibition of intestinal calcium absorption. Initially HARRISON and HARRISON reported that glucocorticoid administration will suppress intestinal calcium transport as measured in vitro by the everted sac technique (HARRISON and HARRISON, 1960). This observation has been confirmed (KIMBERG, 1969; KIMBERG et al., 1971) and is thought to represent one of the mechanisms by which glucocorticoids can suppress hypercalcemia. The mechanism of this suppression has come under investigation, and KIMBERG and colleagues have concluded that the glucocorticoids do not affect intestinal calcium absorption by affecting vitamin D metabolism (FAVUS et al., 1973a, b). In support of this conclusion, 1,25-$(OH)_2D_3$ from exogenous sources can only partially overcome the intestinal calcium absorption suppression brought about by the glucocorticoids (FAVUS et al., 1973b). On the other hand, CARRE et al. (1974) reported that glucocorticoids bring about a conversion of 1,25-$(OH)_2D_3$ to a closely migrating but inactive metabolite. They suggest that the glucocorticoids suppress intestinal calcium absorption by facilitating the further conversion of 1,25-$(OH)_2D_3$ to an inactive product. Attempts to reproduce this work in our own laboratory have not been fruitful, so the question of how the glucocorticoids affect intestinal calcium absorption remains to be answered.

It has been reported that prolactin and growth hormone increase intestinal calcium transport (SPANOS and MACINTYRE, 1977). The mechanism of this phenomenon remains unknown except that recent results suggest that prolactin may stimulate the 25-OH-D_3-1-hydroxylase, which may indicate that the mechanism involves a systemic elevation of 1,25-$(OH)_2D_3$, which would in turn stimulate intestinal calcium transport.

3. The Molecular Mechanism of Action of 1,25-$(OH)_2D_3$ in Intestinal Calcium Transport

During the course of discovery of the vitamin D metabolites, repeated attempts at studying the subcellular location of vitamin D in the intestine have appeared. One of the earliest reports is by HAUSSLER and NORMAN (1967) in which they reported that the nuclear fraction contained some 90 percent of the tissue radioactivity arising from radioactive vitamin D. They concluded that this activity is entirely as unchanged vitamin D_3. Shortly thereafter STOHS and DELUCA (1967) reported that the nuclear-debris fraction possesses a major portion of the radioactivity derived from radioactive vitamin D. They demonstrated that the radioactivity was found entirely in the polar metabolite fractions, which was then called peak 4 and which included not only 25-OH-D_3 but also the 1,25-$(OH)_2D_3$. Following the isolation and identification of 25-OH-D_3, HAUSSLER et al. (1968) reported that intestinal chromatin contains a metabolite more polar than 25-OH-D_3. Similar results were reported by LAWSON, WILSON and KODICEK in which they demonstrated the appearance of a metabolite termed peak P in the intestinal nuclei from rachitic chicks given 1α-^{3}H and 4-^{14}C vitamin D_3 (LAWSON et al., 1969). However, the chromatin isolation method used by HAUSSLER et al. yielded preparations that were far from homogeneous (CHEN et al., 1970). When chromatin was isolated by the method of MARUSHIGE and BONNER, yielding homogenous chromatin, much less of the radioactivity could be found associated with this fraction (CHEN et al., 1970). It was at this time that 1,25-$(OH)_2D_3$ was isolated and chemically identified as 1,25-$(OH)_2D_3$ (HOLICK et al., 1971a, b). Following this event, CHEN and DELUCA reexamined the question of subcellular location of radioactive 1,25-$(OH)_2D_3$ (CHEN et al., 1970). Again 80–90 percent of the radioactivity from 1,25-$(OH)_2D_3$ was found associated with the nuclear-debris fraction. Using the best methods of isolating pure nuclei, only 20 percent of the total homogenate DNA from intestine could be isolated as pure nuclei. This pure fraction accounted for only 20 percent of the total homogenate radioactivity. Chromatin isolated by the method of MARUSHIGE and BONNER also revealed only 20 percent of the cellular radioactivity in pure chromatin. LAWSON also obtained similar results in his attempts at obtaining pure chromatin (LAWSON and WILSON, 1974). Thus the question of the subcellular location of 1,25-$(OH)_2D_3$ was never totally resolved. Recently it has been possible to synthesize chemically radioactive 25-OH-D_3 of extremely high specific activity (80–100 Ci/mmol) (YAMADA et al., 1978). This substance, when given in vivo and when studied in frozen sections of intestine, was specifically localized in the nuclei of the villus cells and crypt cells (Fig. 10) (ZILE et al., 1978). It appeared in the nuclei at about 2–2½ h postinjection, reached a maximum at 4 h postinjection, and was still present in high levels 6 h after administration. In the chick maximal intestinal calcium absorption in response to this dose of 1,25-$(OH)_2D_3$ was found at 9 h. No specific nuclear location could be found in skeletal muscle, smooth muscle, liver, large sections of the kidney, or parathyroid glands. Unfortunately the results of bone autoradiography with these truly physiologic doses are not yet available. However, we can now say with confidence that in vivo the location of 1,25-$(OH)_2D_3$ prior to the initiation of intestinal calcium transport is the nuclei of small intestinal villus cells and the nuclei of intestinal crypt cells.

Inasmuch as vitamin D is similar to the steroid it is natural to assume that 1,25-$(OH)_2D_3$ might function in a manner similar to the mechanism believed to be the case for the steroid (O'MALLEY and MCGUIRE, 1968). Thus it might be suspected that 1,25-$(OH)_2D_3$ might become associated with a cytoplasmic receptor which would then be transferred to the nucleus and in some unknown manner effect the transcription of specific genomes which would code for calcium and phosphorus transport proteins. BRUMBAUGH and HAUSSLER provided the first evidence for the existence of a receptor protein for 1,25-$(OH)_2D_3$ in the cytoplasm from rachitic chick intestine (BRUMBAUGH and HAUSSLER, 1973; 1974a). In a series of papers they described the existence of a 3.0S cytosol receptor that then

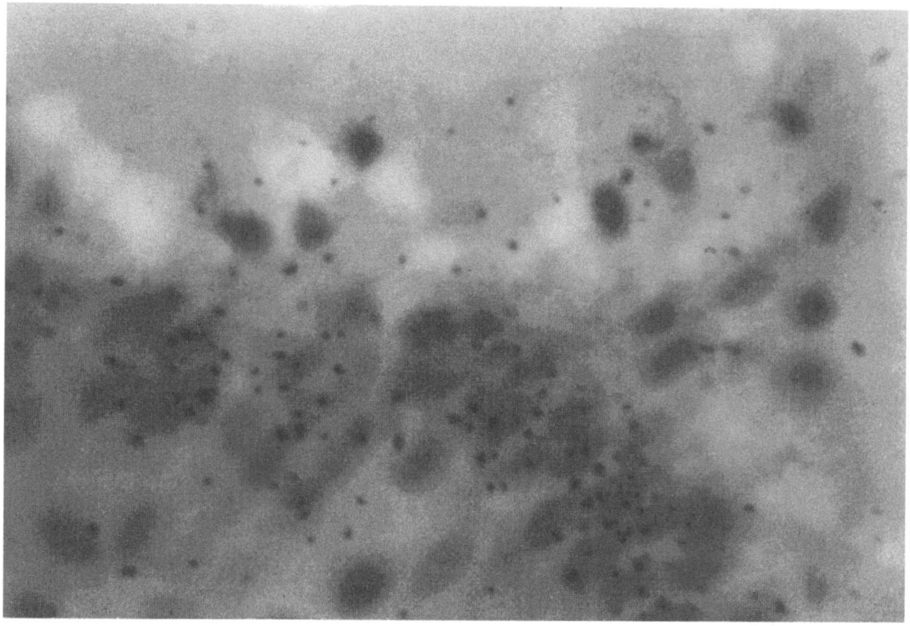

Fig. 10. The subcellular localization of ^3H-labeled 1,25-$(OH)_2D_3$ in the small intestine of the chick prior to initiation of intestinal calcium transport. Rachitic chickens were given a single injection of 650 pmol or 50 μCi of 1,25-$(OH)_2$[23,24-^3H]D_3. Two and one-half hours later, intestinal mucosa was harvested from the duodenum and submitted to frozen tissue sectioning. Autoradiography was performed to reveal the location of the tritium. The specific nuclear location was noted in intestinal mucosa as shown in the figure, but not in the submucosa, smooth muscle, skeletal muscle, heart muscle, liver, and glomerulus of the kidney. Other specific localization was found in the osteoblasts of bone, osteocytes, chondrocytes, and in certain tubule cells of the kidney

becomes bound to nuclear chromatin when the mixture of cytosol plus intestinal chromatin is warmed to 37 °C (BRUMBAUGH and HAUSSLER, 1974b). The transfer to chromatin is specific to intestinal cytosol since it is not carried out by cytosol from other tissues. Although the bare outlines of this mechanism appear, much remains to be done. In fact, the existence of a specific 1,25-$(OH)_2D_3$-binding protein in the cytosol of rats and of chicks could not be confirmed at first (KREAM et al., 1976). However, extensive washing of the intestinal mucosa to eliminate proteolytic activity helped considerably in demonstrating the existence of a specific 1,25-$(OH)_2D_3$ protein in intestinal cytosol from rachitic chi :ks. Furthermore, it has been found that high salt concentrations and the presence of a sulfhydryl protecting group such as dithiothreitol were very effective in permitting the demonstration of the cytosol receptors (KREAM et al., 1977a). It is now clear that a highly specific binding protein in the cytosol of rachitic chicks can be readily demonstrated, and its sedimentation coefficient is 3.7S (KREAM et al., 1977a). This protein is highly specific for 1,25-$(OH)_2D_3$, and can be competed for by a 10–100-fold excess of 1,24(R),25-$(OH)_3D_3$, a 100-fold excess of 1α-OH-D_3, or 1,000-fold excess of 25-OH-D_3 (KREAM et al., 1977b; EISMAN and DELUCA, 1977). The high degree of specificity of this cytosol receptor is illustrated in Fig.

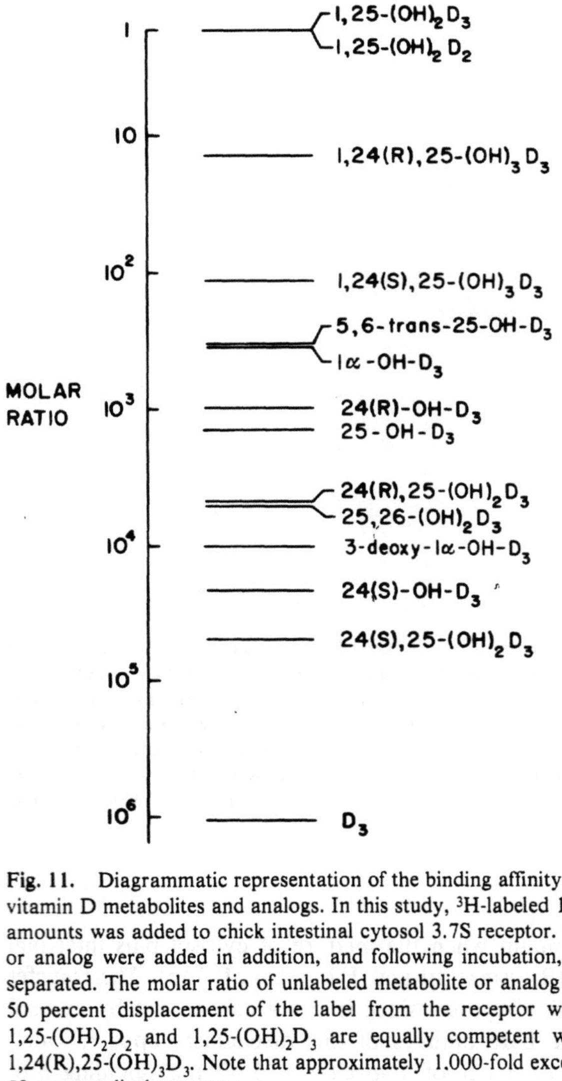

Fig. 11. Diagrammatic representation of the binding affinity of chick intestinal cytosol for the various vitamin D metabolites and analogs. In this study, ^{3}H-labeled 1,25-$(OH)_2D_3$ in approximately saturating amounts was added to chick intestinal cytosol 3.7S receptor. Varying amounts of unlabeled metabolite or analog were added in addition, and following incubation, the protein-bound and free tritium were separated. The molar ratio of unlabeled metabolite or analog to the labeled 1,25-$(OH)_2D_3$ required for 50 percent displacement of the label from the receptor was calculated and is plotted. Note that 1,25-$(OH)_2D_2$ and 1,25-$(OH)_2D_3$ are equally competent whereas the nearest other competitor is 1,24(R),25-$(OH)_3D_3$. Note that approximately 1.000-fold excess of 25-OH-D_3 is required to produce a 50 percent displacement

11, which shows the relative concentration of unlabeled analog that is required to provide 50 percent competition for binding site on the chick intestinal cytosol protein (EISMAN and DELUCA, 1977). In the rat there appears to be a 3.2S cytosol protein which is highly specific for 1,25-$(OH)_2D_3$ (KREAM et al., 1977a). There exists in the cytosol preparations of a large variety of tissues a 6S binding protein specific for 25-OH-D_3 (KREAM et al., 1977b). This 6S component does not appear in cells that have been isolated free of plasma protein (VANBAELEN et al., 1977; KREAM and DELUCA, unpublished results). The plasma transport protein for vitamin D and its metabolites have a sedimentation value of 4.1S. Thus the 6S protein did not appear to be the cytoplasmic 3.2S receptor or plasma transport protein. However, when plasma transport protein is added to intestinal cytosol, a 4.1S binder is not observed but instead a 6S peak is observed. It has also been demonstrated that the 6S cytosol material is immunologically identical to the plasma transport protein but not the 3.2S cytosol receptor (KREAM and DELUCA, unpublished results). Furthermore, VANBAELEN and associates have provided firm evidence that the 6S cytosol binder for 25-OH-D_3 represents an artifactual interaction between the 4.1S plasma protein and an unknown nonspecific cytosol protein (VANBAELEN et al., 1977). The 6S component can be heated to 60 °C yielding once again the stable 4.1S plasma transport protein and destroying the cytosol material that binds to the 4.1S protein. In any case the 6S "protein" is found in a large variety of tissues (HADDAD and BIRGE, 1975), which strongly suggests that it cannot be a specific receptor protein. The results of VANBAELEN and those from our own group are consistent with this concept.

The 3.7S cytosol protein from rachitic chick plasma has been utilized in the development of a specific 1,25-$(OH)_2D_3$ competitive protein-binding assay (EISMAN et al., 1976a, b). This assay involves extraction with dichloromethane, purification of the 1,25-$(OH)_2D_3$ on a Sephadex LH-20 column developed in a solvent system of 90 parts chloroform, 10 parts Skellysolve B, and 10 parts methanol. The 1,25-$(OH)_2D_3$ portion of the peak is then subjected to high-pressure liquid chromatography on fine-grain silicic acid columns with a solvent system of 10 percent isopropanol in hexane. The 1,25-$(OH)_2D_3$ substance is then measured by competitive intestinal receptor binding assay. This assay is reasonably convenient, accurate, and sensitive with the high specific activity 1,25-$(OH)_2D_3$ (80 Ci/mmol) to very low values of 1–2 pg. BRUMBAUGH and HAUSSLER have developed a chromatin-binding assay which utilizes the cytosol-binding protein and intestinal chromatin in a manner similar to the cytosol-binding assay described above. The results of these two assays agree very well with each other and also agree with a bone tissue-culture bioassay developed by STERN et al. (1977). A typical competitive binding assay curve is shown in Fig. 12. A detailed discussion of this method of assay is inappropriate for this review and readers are referred to the original papers for details.

To summarize the current state of the art in this area, Fig. 13 contains a diagram of the presumed molecular mechanism of action of 1,25-$(OH)_2D_3$ in the stimulation of intestinal calcium transport. In this case the chick intestinal villus cell is depicted. It is believed that 1,25-$(OH)_2D_3$ transported on the 4.1S plasma transport protein is transferred to the villus cell where it becomes associated with a 3.7S cytosol receptor protein. This receptor protein becomes modified and enters the nucleus where it interacts with the nuclear chromatin in some unknown fashion, bringing about transcription of specific genes that code for the calcium and phosphorus transport systems. Increased DNA template activity has already been demonstrated in response to vitamin D (HALLICK and DELUCA, 1969) and more recently in response to 1,25-$(OH)_2D_3$ (ZERWEKH et al., 1976) consistent with the idea that the receptor protein 1,25-$(OH)_2D_3$ complex unmasks specific genes which then become subject to transcriptase activity. The mRNAs that code for the transport proteins are then translated into specific proteins (which are unknown at the present time) that make their appearance at the brush border surface. There, by an unknown mechanism, calcium is permitted to enter

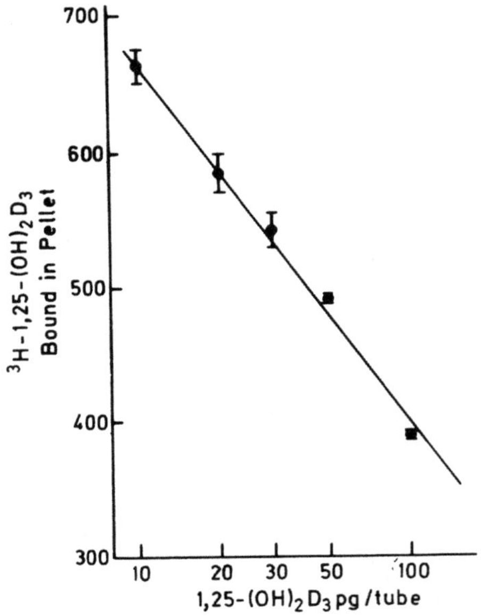

Fig. 12. Standard curve in the competitive cytosol receptor-protein-binding assay for 1,25-$(OH)_2D_3$. Varying amounts of unlabeled 1,25-$(OH)_2D_3$ were added to the cytosol receptor with approximately saturating amounts of ^3H-labeled 1,25-$(OH)_2D_3$. After incubation for 1 h at 20 °C, the bound from free was separated by polyethylene glycol precipitation of the receptor complex and the amount of bound ^3H-labeled 1,25-$(OH)_2D_3$ is plotted versus the amount of unlabeled 1,25-$(OH)_2D_3$ added

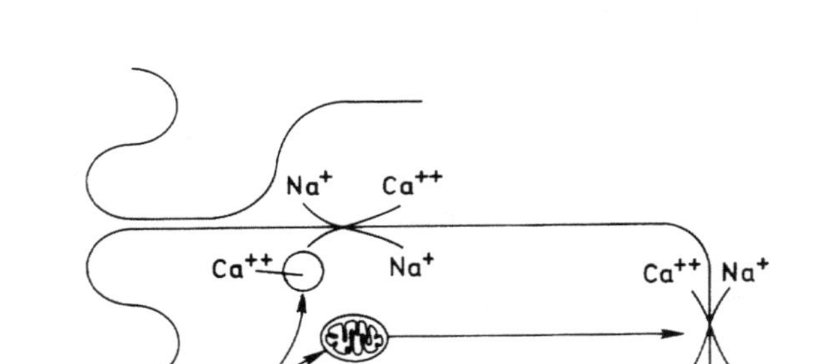

Fig. 13. Diagrammatic representation of the expected mechanism whereby 1,25-$(OH)_2D_3$ initiates intestinal calcium transport in chick intestinal mucosa. Note that 1,25-$(OH)_2D_3$ is believed to interact with a 3.7S cytosol receptor that is then transferred to the nucleus where it, in some unknown manner, initiates transcription of genes that code for calcium transport proteins. These proteins appear presumably at the brush border surface, permitting calcium to enter the intestinal epithelium absorption cells. Calcium is then either packaged in vesicles at the terminal web region, or is taken up by mitochondria. Calcium is expelled from the cell by a sodium-dependent process

the cell where it is either packaged in vesicular membranes near the terminal web of the microvilli or is accepted as calcium phosphate granules in mitochondria. These are then transferred to the basal lateral membrane where calcium is expelled, presumably in a sodium-dependent process. As one can readily surmise, much of this mechanism remains unknown and much of it is speculation. However, at least some progress is being made and it seems likely that the mechanism whereby vitamin D stimulates intestinal calcium absorption will be understood in the next decade or so.

4. Intestinal Phosphate Transport

Although NICOLAYSEN originally believed that phosphate transport was not influenced by vitamin D (NICOLAYSEN, 1937d), HARRISON and HARRISON (1961) demonstrated by the everted sac technique that vitamin D does influence intestinal phosphate transport. Although they were unable to dissociate completely the role of vitamin D in calcium transport from that in phosphate transport, subsequent workers have provided clear evidence that this is the case (CHEN et al., 1974; KOWARSKI and SCHACHTER, 1969; TAYLOR and WASSERMAN, 1972; TAYLOR, 1974b). Sodium is required for phosphate transport at the brush border surface in contrast to the calcium transport mechanism (TAYLOR, 1974b). In addition to this, phosphate transport is most noticeable in the distal segments of the small intestine where the calcium transport mechanism is lower. It is likely that phosphate transport occurs through the entire length of small intestine, but it is most conveniently studied in the distal ileum. Nephrectomy prevents response of intestinal phosphate transport to 25-OH-D_3 but not to 1,25-$(OH)_2D_3$ (CHEN et al., 1974). Finally, WALLING has recently provided evidence that phosphate is transported against an electrochemical potential gradient in response to 1,25-$(OH)_2D_3$ (WALLING, 1977). Little is known concerning the mechanism of phosphate transport, and remains to be studied in detail.

5. Stimulation of Intestinal Calcium Transport by Phosphate Deprivation

CARLSSON first discovered that phosphate deprived animals have high rates of intestinal calcium absorption (CARLSSON, 1953). This finding was confirmed and extended by the work of MORRISSEY and WASSERMAN (1971) and more recently was confirmed by TANAKA et al. (1973b). In addition, BAYLINK and his colleagues provided evidence that phosphate depletion not only stimulates intestinal calcium absorption but also greatly increases the resorption of bone (THOMPSON et al., 1975). As pointed out earlier, phosphate depletion markedly stimulates the elevation of plasma levels of 1,25-$(OH)_2D_3$ by increasing its biogenesis and by decreasing its turnover or increasing its accumulation in both plasma and intestine (TANAKA and DELUCA, 1973; RIBOVICH and DELUCA, 1978b). In animals given 1,25-$(OH)_2D_3$, phosphate depletion nevertheless stimulates intestinal calcium absorption. It therefore appears that phosphate depletion has some effect other than increasing the plasma level of 1,25-$(OH)_2D_3$. Direct measurements have revealed that the intestines of phosphate-depleted animals accumulate more 1,25-$(OH)_2D_3$ than animals maintained on normal phosphate diets (RIBOVICH and DELUCA, 1978b). It appears possible, therefore, that phosphate depletion not only alters the metabolism of 1,25-$(OH)_2D_3$, but it also may alter the target tissue receptiveness to this hormone.

II. Functions of Vitamin D in Bone

1. Mineralization

The very basis for the discovery of vitamin D is the failure of mineralization that results from vitamin D deficiency. It is well known that an absence of vitamin D leads to rickets in the young and osteomalacia in the adult. In young animals and children, two types of bone growths are known. Long bones especially elongate by a process known as endochondral bone formation. In this process, the epiphyseal plate cartilage elongates by a proliferation of the resting chondrocytes. These cells mature into hypertrophic cartilage cells and at this stage have prepared their organic matrix for mineralization. Mineral is then deposited on the matrix giving rise to what is known as endochondral calcification. The hypertrophic cells then die off and are replaced by invading osteoblasts. The calcified chondrocyte-elaborated matrix is resorbed and in its place is elaborated the organic matrix and mineral of newly forming bone. This is accompanied by invasion of the blood vessels, ultimately giving rise to what is known as trabecular bone. In this manner, long bones elongate. In addition to this growth, intramembranous bone formation also occurs that does not involve chondroblast-mediated calcification. Instead, osteoblasts form a membrane of cells which then elaborate organic matrix followed by the mineralization process. The shaping of bones follows a modeling process in which there is bone resorption and mineralization on both the endosteal and periosteal surfaces of bone (FROST, 1966). Again calcification of newly laid down organic matrix elaborated by osteoblasts results. In all cases of vitamin D deficiency, the newly laid down organic matrix of the osteoblasts as well as that of the chondrocytes fails to mineralize. In adults where the growth plate or epiphyseal growth has ceased thus eliminating the endochondral calcification mechanism, only bone remodeling occurs. In this process, bone is resorbed in what is known as resorption cavities or Howship's lacuna, and these lacunas are then filled in by osteoblastic activity. This remodeling process is one that involves activation of cells to resorb the bone; this is mandatorily coupled to the appearance of osteoblasts which then form new bone, giving a three-step sequence of activation of cells for resorption followed by the formation of the resorption cavity which is in turn followed by the elaboration of newly formed bone, termed the formation process (FROST, 1966). Undoubtedly the formation of new bone by the osteoblasts in the remodeling process fails in vitamin D deficiency, thus giving a prolonged total remodeling period and giving rise to large osteoid seams. The failure of mineralization of bone thereby produces rickets in children that is characterized primarily by the widened epiphyseal plate including dyplasia and the rachitic deformations (HESS, 1929; SEBRELL and HARRIS, 1971).

Osteomalacic bone is weak and there may be obvious radiologic evidence of failure of mineralization and fractures. Several theories have been proposed concerning the molecular and cellular events in mineralization (GLIMCHER, 1959; ANDERSON, 1969, 1976; ANDERSON and SAJDERA, 1976). A review of these processes is not appropriate for this monograph. However, it is clear that some phase of this process fails in vitamin D deficiency. The major reason for failure of mineralization is the insufficient supply of calcium and phosphorus to the chondroblasts and osteoblasts that mediate mineralization of newly formed matrix. Whether there is in addition a failure of the mineralization process directly because of the absence of vitamin D metabolites remains largely unknown. There is little doubt that 1,25-$(OH)_2D_3$ does bring about mineralization of bone; whether it is entirely normal or adequate remains to be determined. There have been proposals that 25-OH-D_3 and 24,25-$(OH)_2D_3$ play a functional role in the mineralization process (BORDIER et al., 1971; 1977). Although evidence for this hypothesis is lacking, there may be a role for vitamin D directly in the mineralization process at the osteoblast and/or chondrocyte.

2. Bone Calcium Mobilization

Throughout the course of vitamin D investigation, emphasis has been placed on the mineralization of bone as the possible site of vitamin D action. However, CARLSSON in 1952 provided convincing evidence that vitamin D plays yet another role in bone, namely, in the mobilization of calcium from bone to the extracellular fluid compartment (CARLSSON, 1952; BAUER et al., 1955). It had long been known that vitamin D deficiency results in hypocalcemic tetany (HESS, 1929). Much of this could be rationalized by failure of intestinal calcium absorption. However, this rationale was insufficient to provide an explanation for the results of CARLSSON. Following the discovery of CARLSSON, NICOLAYSEN and EEG-LARSEN (1956) reexamined the question of whether calcium could come from bone in support of serum calcium concentration. It is indeed obvious in animals placed on a calcium-free diet that vitamin D will bring about an elevation of plasma calcium concentration and that the source of this calcium must be from the bone fluid compartment. Recognizing that bone mineral is not in direct communication with the extracellular fluid compartment and that there must be a bone fluid compartment including a hydration layer on the hydroxyapatite crystals, there must be a membrane of cells separating the bone fluid compartment from the extracellular fluid compartment (TALMAGE, 1969). It appears that vitamin D must function at the bone cell membrane to control the flux of calcium from the bone fluid compartment into the extracellular fluid compartment. Vitamin D shares this function with the parathyroid hormone (GARABEDIAN et al., 1974), and, in fact, recent work has demonstrated that mobilization of calcium from the bone fluid compartment requires both parathyroid hormone and 1,25-$(OH)_2D_3$ (GARABEDIAN et al., 1974).

It is therefore clear that under physiologic circumstances the utilization of calcium from bone requires both of these hormonal agents. This function is not to be misconstrued or intermingled with the possible function of these two hormones in directing bone remodeling. Bone remodeling is not responsible for the maintenance of plasma calcium concentration but rather is charged with the responsibility of rebuilding bone primarily to correct microfractures or to maintain a strong and healthy bone. The introduction of organ culture techniques for the study of resorption of bone in vitro has caused considerable confusion with the in vivo generated data concerning calcium homeostasis. Both parathyroid hormone and 1,25-$(OH)_2D_3$ stimulate resorption of bone in culture. It appears that the majority of this bone resorption is osteoclast mediated and that the responses in culture are quite slow relative to the calcium homeostatic responses observed in vivo (RAISZ et al., 1972). It indeed seems possible that the bone culture systems might well represent an initial event in bone modeling or remodeling and may not be related to the calcium homeostatic system. Exactly what the bone organ cultures are measuring remains uncertain, but nevertheless this technique has provided an important insight regarding the role of these two hormones in bone.

Little is known concerning the mechanism of bone resorption in culture in response to these two hormones. The parathyroid hormone responses probably involve cyclic AMP, and the role of 1,25-$(OH)_2D_3$ in these systems probably involves new protein synthesis (TANAKA and DELUCA, 1971). Little is known beyond these two hypotheses. In the case of bone calcium mobilization or calcium homeostasis even less is known.

KODICEK and his colleagues (WEBER et al., 1971), showed that 1,25-$(OH)_2D_3$ is found in the nuclei of bone cells. However, this again was by means of isolation of bone cells and the isolation of nuclei by biochemical techniques. Autoradiography using high-specific-activity 1,25-$(OH)_2D_3$ and frozen sections of bone have not yet been completed. Thus the nuclear location remains a likely but tenuous conclusion.

The mobilization of calcium from bone in support of serum calcium concentration in response to 1,25-$(OH)_2D_3$ is blocked by the prior administration of actinomycin D and other protein synthesis inhibitors (TANAKA and DELUCA, 1971). The administration of actinomycin D after 1,25-$(OH)_2D_3$ does not block this response, consistent with the idea that an early event involving transcription of DNA is involved in the bone calcium mobilization system. The calcium-binding protein of WASSERMAN and TAYLOR has not been found in bone; therefore, no protein is known in bone that is formed in response to 1,25-$(OH)_2D_3$. Obviously much remains to be done in studying this calcium homeostatic mechanism and the responses to 1,25-$(OH)_2D_3$.

3. Other Possible Roles of Vitamin D in Bone

Besides the mineralization process and the processes of bone resorption or bone remodeling and the mobilization of calcium from bone for calcium homeostatic mechanisms, one additional role of vitamin D in the bone has been suggested. Three groups have provided evidence that vitamin D may play a role in the biosynthesis and maturation of collagen in preparation for mineralization (BARNES et al., 1973; RUSSELL and AVIOLI, 1975; GONNERMAN et al., 1976). In the absence of vitamin D, there appears to be inadequate cross-linking of collagen, perhaps the result of inadequate activity of lysyl oxidase, which oxidizes the ε-amino groups of lysine and other amino acids in preparation for Shiff-base condensation for collagen cross-linking. Whether this phenomenon is a direct effect of vitamin D or its metabolites or whether it is the result of changes in mineral homeostasis remains to be determined. At the present time it cannot be regarded as a major function of vitamin D.

III. Kidney

Since 1941 attention has been focused on a possible role of vitamin D in renal handling of calcium and phosphorus. HARRISON and HARRISON (1941) suggested that vitamin D might have a function in improving renal reabsorption of phosphorus. The early experiments of this group were carried out with intact animals and vitamin D administration undoubtedly prompted a suppression of parathyroid hormone secretion which then suppressed parathyroid hormone-mediated phosphaturia. Following the discovery of the vitamin D metabolites, attempts have been made to demonstrate that vitamin D might improve renal reabsorption of phosphorus. Almost all of these experiments were carried out in animals that were not vitamin D deficient and that were manipulated in some manner or other to prove a degree of phosphaturia that could be influenced by the vitamin D metabolites (PUSCHETT et al., 1972; POPOVTZER et al., 1974). This controversial area has not been entirely resolved, although current evidence suggests that vitamin D metabolites do not improve renal reabsorption of phosphorus directly (STEELE et al., 1975). On the other hand, attention has been focused on the possibility that vitamin D, like parathyroid hormone, improves renal reabsorption of calcium. Work by GRAN demonstrated that vitamin D could improve retention of injected calcium in dogs (GRAN, 1960). More recently, however, SUTTON et al. (1977) showed that vitamin D, like parathyroid hormone, improves renal reabsorption of calcium. It must be recognized, however, that 99 percent of the filtered calcium is reabsorbed in the absence of vitamin D or parathyroid hormone in any case (KLEEMAN et al., 1961). However, the remaining 1 percent could provide a significant fraction of calcium if one considers that man filters in the neighborhood of 7–10 g of calcium per day (NORDIN and SMITH, 1965). The site of vitamin D action on renal reabsorption of calcium is unknown, although the best evidence suggests that it is in the distal tubule.

One of the most significant breakthroughs in the functions of vitamin D and its metabolites has been provided by BONJOUR et al. (1977). In a thorough study of phosphate reabsorption this group examined the phosphate handling of animals having slight hyperphosphatemia. Rather than demonstrating a role of 1,25-$(OH)_2D_3$ in renal reabsorption of phosphorus, they demonstrated that 1,25-$(OH)_2D_3$ under conditions of adequate or more than adequate circulating phosphate stimulates phosphaturia. It seemed clear from their results that the parathyroid hormone might sustain phosphaturia by increasing the renal synthesis of 1,25-$(OH)_2D_3$. However, it is certain that parathyroid hormone directly blocks renal tubular phosphate reabsorption, thereby giving rise to phosphaturia in its own right. However, it appears that the presence of 1,25-$(OH)_2D_3$ does influence renal handling of phosphate, resulting in phosphaturia under conditions of phosphate loading or hyperphosphatemia. The nature of this mechanism is not understood and may well be indirect because of the period of time required for the response.

VI. The Function of Vitamin D in Muscle and Elsewhere

From the clinical world has come the observation that patients suffering from rickets or osteomalacia demonstrate extreme muscle weakness and lack of muscle tone (HESS, 1929; SEBRELL and HARRIS, 1971; REED et al., 1939). One of the early results of vitamin D administration is an improvement in muscle strength. This has led to the suggestion that vitamin D must play a role in muscle either directly or indirectly. KODICEK reported that vitamin D accumulates in the sarcolemma of muscle, but these results were obtained with pharmacologic doses of radioactive vitamin D. With physiologic amounts of vitamin D, large amounts of the vitamin can be found in the muscle mass (NORMAN and DELUCA, 1963; KODICEK, 1960). However, it is not concentrated in that tissue but may be there simply because of the large amount of membrane represented by the muscle mass. In any case these results have prompted an investigation by BIRGE and HADDAD into a possible role of the vitamin D metabolites in muscle (BIRGE and HADDAD, 1975). Although they have reported changes in ATP synthesis and possibly amino acid incorporation, these results are not yet convincing. It seems likely that if vitamin D is involved in muscle function, it is probably at the level of calcium and phosphorus transfer reactions into muscle cells or muscle subcellular components. BIRGE and HADDAD, on the basis of the widespread distribution of the 6S cytosol binder for 25-OH-D_3, have postulated a generalized role for this metabolite in support of growth and tissue proliferation (HADDAD et al., 1973b). Although it has long been known that vitamin D improves growth of animals, it is not clear whether the growth stimulation found with vitamin D is a direct or indirect effect of changes in mineral metabolism. In fact, STEENBOCK and HERTING noted that under conditions of hypocalcemia, vitamin D stimulates growth, whereas in animals given high dietary levels of calcium, vitamin D may actually inhibit growth (STEENBOCK and HERTING, 1955). It seems likely that the growth responses to vitamin D are the result of changes in mineral metabolism.

Finally, some mention should be made of the possible role of vitamin D in regulation of parathyroid hormone secretion. The discovery of the vitamin D metabolites and of its intimate interrelationship with parathyroid hormone function has led to the suggestion that vitamin D may be involved in the regulation of parathyroid hormone secretion (OLDHAM et al., 1974). The discovery of a calcium-binding protein in parathyroid glands that later did not appear to be vitamin D dependent (OLDHAM et al., 1974) supported this idea. In any case, HENRY and NORMAN (1975) reported that parathyroid glands specifically accumulate 1,25-$(OH)_2D_3$ in a manner similar to that in the intestine. HAUSSLER's and HADDAD's groups both reported the presence of a 1,25-$(OH)_2D_3$-binding protein specific for that metabolite in parathyroid tissue (BRUMBAUGH et al., 1975; HADDAD et al., 1976). Beyond that, several investigators have attempted to show that 1,25-$(OH)_2D_3$ either stimulates or suppresses parathyroid hormone secretion. The results that have been obtained are diverse and controversial. CHERTOW reports that parathyroid hormone secretion is suppressed by 1,25-$(OH)_2D_3$ (CHERTOW et al., 1975), while others could find either no difference or a stimulation of secretion. This area remains controversial and so far has not yet been resolved. An additional twist was provided by HENRY and NORMAN, who suggested that 24,25-$(OH)_2D_3$ together with 1,25-$(OH)_2D_3$ suppresses parathyroid gland size (HENRY et al., 1977). They postulated that these forms of vitamin D working in concert may well regulate parathyroid hormone secretion. This indirect measure of parathyroid hormone function is not sufficiently definitive to provide firm evidence. Studies on the role of 24,25-$(OH)_2D_3$ and parathyroid hormone secretion have likewise been of an unexpected and controversial nature. Thus, the possible role of the vitamin D metabolites in regulation of parathyroid hormone secretion remains unresolved at this writing.

G. Analogs of 1,25-Dihydroxyvitamin D_3 and 25-Hydroxyvitamin D_3

(Fig. 14)

I. Analogs of 25-Hydroxyvitamin D_3

Following the discovery of 25-OH-D_3 interest has been generated in analogs of vitamin D possessing the 25-hydroxyl function. In a sense the dihydrotachysterols, the 5,6-trans-25-OH-D_3, and the isotachysterols discussed above can be considered as analogs of either 25-OH-D_3 or 1,25-$(OH)_2D_3$. Because of the rotation of ring A about the 5,6 double bond, these compounds assume the role of analogs of 1,25-$(OH)_2D_3$ especially since they cannot be 1-hydroxylated by the 1-hydroxylase of the kidney. It is sufficient to reaffirm that these compounds, although effective in the absence of kidneys, are very poor analogs of 1,25-$(OH)_2D_3$, being less than 1/1,000 as active as

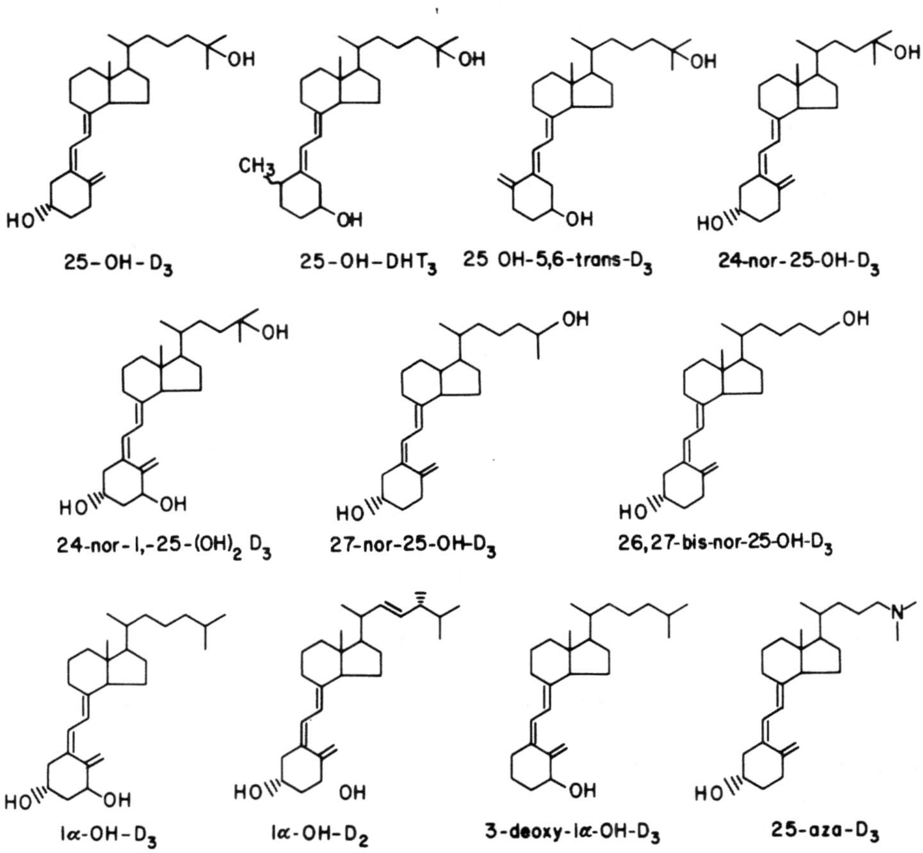

Fig. 14. Analogs of 1,25-$(OH)_2D_3$ which are of current interest in our understanding of the metabolism and function of the vitamin

1,25-$(OH)_2D_3$. The dihydrotachysterols are of some interest because they represent a commercially available substitute for 1,25-$(OH)_2D_3$ in the treatment of renal osteodystrophy, hypoparathyroidism, and other diseases where there is defective absorption and utilization of calcium.

24-Nor, 27-nor, and 26,27-bisnor-25-OH-D_3 have all been prepared and have very limited biological activity of the order of 1/1,000 that of vitamin D. This low activity is not the result of failure of 1-hydroxylation since the 5,6-trans isomers provide little increase in activity, and 24-nor-1,25-$(OH)_2D_3$ has low levels of activity (HOLICK et al., 1975a). The report that the latter compound is an antivitamin has appeared, but requires additional confirmation before it can be accepted (JOHNSON et al., 1975).

II. 1α-Hydroxyvitamin D_3 and 1α-Hydroxyvitamin D_2

With the discovery of 1,25-$(OH)_2D_3$ came attempts at chemical synthesis. During the course of development of methods for introduction of the 1-hydroxyl function into the sterol precursors of vitamin D, it was possible to synthesize 1α-hydroxycholesterol (HOLICK et al., 1973b). This was converted to the 5,7-diene and subsequently to the vitamin, giving one of the most important analogs of 1,25-$(OH)_2D_3$, namely, 1α-OHD_3 (HOLICK et al., 1973b). This form of vitamin D_3 was found to be about ½ as active as 1,25-$(OH)_2D_3$ in the rat (HOLICK et al., 1975) and almost equally active to 1,25-$(OH)_2D_3$ in the chick (HAUSSLER et al., 1973). In man it proves to be approximately ½ as active as 1,25-$(OH)_2D_3$ in the treatment of certain metabolic bone diseases (CHAN et al., 1977; NEER et al., 1975; BALSAN et al., 1975). The successful synthesis of 1α-OH-D_3 was followed by the successful synthesis of 1α-OH-D_2 (LAM et al., 1974a). This substance also proved to be about ½ as active as 1,25-$(OH)_2D_3$ in mammals (REEVE et al., 1978), but was only about 1/10 as active as 1α-OH-D_3 in birds (JONES et al., 1976b), as might be expected in view of the side-chain discrimination against vitamin D metabolites and analogs discussed previously. 1α-OH-D_2 has not yet been studied in man. Of some interest is the fact that 1α-OH-D_2 is considerably less active than 1α-OH-D_3 in the mobilization of calcium from bone, otherwise being equally active to 1α-OH-D_3 in mammals in every other respect (REEVE et al., 1978). Thus this analog is one of the first showing a differential response between processes of intestinal absorption and mineralization and bone mobilization of calcium.

It was of considerable interest whether 1α-OH-D_3 acted directly without 25-hydroxylation, which would suggest that 25-hydroxylation was only necessary for recognition by the 1-hydroxylase enzyme system. However, with the chemical synthesis of tritiated 1α-OH-D_3 by two groups (HOLICK et al., 1976a; TOHIRA et al., 1977), it was possible to demonstrate clearly that 1α-OH-D_3 is rapidly converted to 1,25-$(OH)_2D_3$ before it elicits the elevation of intestinal calcium transport or the mobilization of calcium from bone (HOLICK et al., 1976a). Similar conclusions were reached by ZERWEKH et al. using the receptor protein system to analyze for 1,25-$(OH)_2D_3$ (ZERWEKH et al., 1974). Although these results demonstrated that in fact the 1α-OH-D_3 was probably 25-hydroxylated before it carried out its functions in man, the question of whether it can function directly without 25-hydroxylation remained. Recently NAPOLI et al. completed chemical synthesis of 25-fluoro-1α-OH-D_3 (NAPOLI et al., 1977b), which eliminates the possibility of 25-hydroxylation. This compound was found to be about 1/50 as active as 1,25-$(OH)_2D_3$ in vivo but was about equal to 1α-OH-D_3 in the binding to the cytosol receptor protein (NAPOLI et al.). In every respect it appears that the 1α-OH-25-fluoro compound must act without 25-hydroxylation, but it appears that some 50-fold excess of this compound is required to bring about the same response as does 1,25-$(OH)_2D_3$. Thus it appears that 1α-OH-D_3 can act without 25-hydroxylation if provided at 50–100 times the amount of 1,25-$(OH)_2D_3$.

III. 3-Deoxy-1α-Hydroxyvitamin D_3 and 3-Deoxy-1,25-Dihydroxyvitamin D_3

In an attempt to determine whether the 3-hydroxyl function might be insignificant following the introduction of the 25-hydroxy and the 1-hydroxy functions, 3-deoxy-1α-OH-D_3 has been synthesized by two groups (LAM et al., 1974b; OKAMURA et al., 1974a), and 3-deoxy-1α,25-$(OH)_2D_3$ has been synthesized by one group (OKAMURA et al., 1975). OKAMURA and his colleagues suggested that since two conformers of the vitamin D A ring are possible as revealed by nuclear magnetic resonance (nmr) studies, the receptor proteins may be specific for only one of these conformers (OKAMURA et al., 1974b). Thus by removing the 3-hydroxyl, one can force the A ring to be predominantly in one of those conformations resulting in the 1-hydroxyl being in the axial position. OKAMURA and colleagues postulated, therefore, that this compound should have super-vitamin D or super-1,25-$(OH)_2D_3$ activity. In fact these compounds are disappointingly inactive in every respect, being 1/50 as active in binding to the receptor protein and being even less active than that in vivo (ONISKO et al., 1977a). In organ cultures, the 3-deoxy-1α-OH-D_3 is virtually inactive as compared to the 1α-OH-D_3 compound (STERN et al., 1975). Thus the idea of a super-active vitamin D based on the topographic predictions of OKAMURA has not been supported. It is also important to realize that if there is a rapid conformational shift in the A ring in solution as shown by nmr, it seems possible that the receptor would select for the conformer shifting the equilibrium in the direction of the favored conformer. The value of the conformational concept, therefore, remains in serious doubt. The existence of the conformers as demonstrated originally by LAMAR and BUDD (1974) and confirmed by OKAMURA and colleagues (WING et al., 1974), was firmly established by DAHL and colleagues, who were able to crystallize out the two conformers and demonstrate their detailed structure by X-ray crystallography (TRINH-TOAN et al., 1976).

IV. Other Analogs of Vitamin D

Perhaps the only compounds that should be mentioned here are those that represent attempts to obtain an antivitamin D. NORMAN and his colleagues suggested that 24-nor-1α,25-$(OH)_2D_3$ might have antivitamin D activity (JOHNSON et al., 1975). So far this has not been confirmed and remains unknown. Attempts to synthesize an antivitamin D compound have persisted in the author's laboratories. Recently 25-aza-vitamin D_3 has been prepared and shown to block vitamin D metabolism at the 25-hydroxylation stage (ONISKO et al., 1977b). In fact, when given prior to vitamin D_3, this compound can block the effect of a physiologic amount of vitamin D for about 16 h. More frequent injections of the analog can effectively prevent the responses to vitamin D, all of which are consistent with the idea that 25-hydroxylation is arrested. Whether this compound will be of use in control of hypercalcemia or in the study of vitamin D metabolism remains to be determined, however. Somewhere in the neighborhood of 1,000–5,000-fold excess of the 25-aza-vitamin D appears to be necessary to block the physiologic response to vitamin D. Undoubtedly a large number of analogs can be expected in the future in the area of analogs of 1,25-$(OH)_2D_3$, both as antivitamins and as attempts to obtain specialized activity on one organ to the exclusion of activity on other organs.

H. Use of Vitamin D Compounds in Medicine, Especially 1,25-Dihydroxyvitamin D_3

The discovery of the vitamin D metabolites has ushered in a new era in the treatment of metabolic bone disease. Its utility as compared to the peptide hormones, known to play a role in calcium and phosphorus metabolism, lies in the fact that it is a steroid and can be administered orally with longer lasting effectiveness. It might be expected that there are diseases in which there is interference with 25-hydroxylation of vitamin D. So far this has not been clearly demonstrated, although it might be expected that biliary atresia has associated with it inadequate 25-hydroxylation. Phenobarbital and dilantin-induced osteomalacia is likely to be associated with low plasma levels of 25-OH-D_3, which suggests that these drugs may be inducing enzymes that destroy vitamin D and its metabolites (HAHN et al., 1972). This disease can be treated with either increased amounts of vitamin D or specifically with 25-OH-D_3 (HAHN and AVIOLI, 1977). The glucocorticoids have been shown to reduce plasma levels of 25-OH-D_3 (KLEIN et al., 1977), which suggests that the osteoporosis associated with glucocorticoid treatment might be improved or corrected by the administration of either 25-OH-D_3 or 1,25-$(OH)_2D_3$ (KLEIN et al., 1977).

Perhaps the most obivous application of the vitamin D metabolites is in the area of renal osteodystrophy and hypoparathyroidism. In the case of hypoparathyroid patients, it is obvious that these patients cannot increase their biogenesis of 1,25-$(OH)_2D_3$ in response to hypocalcemia. As a result, they have low intestinal calcium absorption and cannot mobilize calcium from bone. Undoubtedly if the patients are truly parathyroid hormone deficient, bone calcium cannot be used as a source of calcium for maintaining serum calcium concentration. On the other hand, 1,25-$(OH)_2D_3$ can be used together with sufficient amounts of dietary calcium to support plasma calcium concentration. This in fact has proved to be an effective approach to therapy of hypoparathyroidism and the related disease, pseudohypoparathyroidism (NEER et al., 1975; KOOH et al., 1975). These diseases also have associated with them low plasma levels of 1,25-$(OH)_2D_3$ (DREZNER et al., 1976; HAUSSLER et al., 1976). In the case of renal osteodystrophy, the major factor in the derangements in calcium metabolism brought about by the disease is a failure to synthesize 1,25-$(OH)_2D_3$. Recent results have revealed that as the glomerular filtration rates of renal failure patients approach 30 or less, the plasma levels of 1,25-$(OH)_2D_3$ become undetectable (SLATOPOLSKY and DELUCA, unpublished results). This leads to low calcium absorption, secondary responses by the parathyroid glands including hypertrophy, and gives secondary hyperparathyroidism, which during the development of the disease brings about rapid erosion or secondary osteitis fibrosa (BRICKER et al., 1969; DELUCA and AVIOLI, 1978). In addition, the lack of 1,25-$(OH)_2D_3$ probably results in osteomalacia. High circulating parathyroid hormone plus lack of 1,25-$(OH)_2D_3$ may be a contributing factor to the osteosclerosis aspect of the disease as well (DELUCA and AVIOLI, 1978). This disease is greatly improved by the administration of 1,25-$(OH)_2D_3$ or one of its analogs (CHAN et al., 1977; SILVERBERG et al., 1975; BRICKMAN et al., 1972; CHESNEY et al., 1978; CHAN et al., 1975; CHAN and DELUCA, 1977; DAVIE et al., 1976; PIERIDES et al., 1976; FOURNIER et al., 1976). This compound will probably be much more useful in preventing the development of the bone disease associated with chronic renal failure, since the secondary hyperparathyroidism can be prevented as can the osteomalacia and probably the osteosclerosis if the patients are given 1,25-$(OH)_2D_3$ as they enter renal failure.

Hypocalcemia of premature infants is another obvious application of 1,25-$(OH)_2D_3$. The basis of hypocalcemic tetany of premature infants and of infants from deprived mothers remains unknown, although at least one report has revealed the utility of 1,25-$(OH)_2D_3$ in preventing this condition (KOOH et al., 1976).

A specific genetic block in vitamin D metabolism has been postulated (FRASER et al., 1973) for vitamin D-dependency rickets, which was discovered by PRADER et al. (1961). In this disease, children present with rickets in the face of normal intakes of vitamin D. The disease can be corrected by giving large amounts of vitamin D, often as high as 100,000 units of vitamin D daily. The basis for the disease was not understood until the elucidation of vitamin D metabolism. 25-OH-D_3 can be used in the treatment of this disease, but pharmacologic amounts of the compound are required, although much less than vitamin D itself (FRASER et al., 1973). However, physiologic amounts of 1,25-$(OH)_2D_3$ can be used effectively (FRASER et al., 1973). Furthermore, plasma levels of 1,25-$(OH)_2D_3$ have been shown to be low in this disease, which confirms the postulation of a metabolic block at the 1-hydroxylation stage of vitamin D (FRASER et al., unpublished results). However, direct measurements of 1-hydroxylase have not been made, which leaves the one remaining link in proving that this is a defect in vitamin D metabolism.

The hypophosphatemic X-linked dominant vitamin D resistant rachitic disease is apparently not a defect in vitamin D metabolism to 1,25-$(OH)_2D_3$ (GLORIEUX et al., 1973; BRICKMAN et al., 1973; O'DOHERTY et al., 1977). Instead, this disease appears to be a block in phosphate transport mechanisms, especially in renal tubular reabsorption of phosphate, giving rise to phosphate wasting and hypophosphatemia (GLORIEUX and SCRIVER, 1972; EICHER et al., 1976). Often there is associated inadequate calcium absorption with normal plasma calcium levels. The disease is treated best by the frequent administration of oral phosphate and the provision of 1,25-$(OH)_2D_3$ to improve intestinal absorption of calcium and prevent secondary hyperparathyroidism (GLORIEUX et al., 1972; HIRSCHMAN et al., 1978; RASMUSSEN et al., 1978). Recent results have revealed that these patients also have lower than normal levels of 1,25-$(OH)_2D_3$ in their plasma (DELUCA, unpublished results), but this is probably secondary to the primary defect in phosphate transport mechanisms.

The major metabolic bone disease that afflicts man in terms of numbers is osteopenia, which is related to the postmenopausal state in the case of women. This loss of bone gives rise to symptomatic bone disease known as osteoporosis or a mixture of osteoporosis and osteomalacia (NORDIN, 1960, 1971; HEANEY, 1977). The metabolic basis for the bone disease remains unknown despite intensive investigation. One contributing factor is the inadequate ability of aging patients to absorb sufficient amounts of calcium to meet their soft tissue needs (Nordin, 1960, 1971; Heaney, 1977; Riggs and Gallagher, 1977). This results in the utilization of skeletal calcium to support plasma calcium concentration, and over a period of years this results in loss of bone mass and osteopenia.

Many factors contribute to the bone disease found in older people. Another factor is inadequate calcium intake or high dietary phosphate intakes (Nordin, 1960, 1971; Heaney, 1977; Riggs and Gallagher 1977). Undoubtedly changes in the sex hormones are involved and in view of the fact that sex hormones may play a role in the regulation of vitamin D metabolism, it is possible that the inadequate biogenesis of 1,25-$(OH)_2D_3$, postulated to take place in osteoporotic patients, may be related to an inadequate supply of sex hormones in the case of postmenopausal women (Tanaka et al., 1976b; Castillo et al., 1977; Nordin, 1960, 1971; Heaney, 1977; Riggs and Gallagher, 1977). In any case the use of the vitamin D metabolites in the treatment of osteoporosis is under study. The exact rationale for their use is unclear, but they may provide some relief from this disease.

Finally, it should be mentioned that 25-OH-D_3, 1α-OH-D_3, and 1,25-$(OH)_2D_3$ are being prepared for use in modern medicine relating to metabolic bone disease. Although the specific need for 25-OH-D_3 appears to be limited, it must be borne in mind that this compound can serve as an analog of 1,25-$(OH)_2D_3$ when given in sufficient amounts. This is explained by the fact that the 1,25-$(OH)_2D_3$ receptor protein will recognize 25-OH-D_3 if present in sufficient concentrations. There are pharmacologic arguments as to why this compound should be used and certainly it represents an improvement over vitamin D therapy that has been used in the past. Vitamin D therapy is faced with the problem of vitamin D toxicity, which is difficult to deal with once it has happened, and the rather slow responses that make management difficult. All three new compounds have much shorter half-lives than vitamin D within the body; hypercalcemia can be readily corrected by merely withdrawing the compound, which provides important new benefits of the use of these compounds in place of standard vitamin D preparations. Hopefully the vitamin D metabolites and analogs will become available very shortly to be utilized where there are clear indications of their benefit.

J. Summary and Conclusions

The field of vitamin D metabolism and function has had an explosive era of new information. We have learned that vitamin D is a precursor of at last one hormone and that the biogenesis of this hormone, which takes place in the kidney, is strongly regulated by the need for calcium or the need for phosphorus. Additionally it can be regulated under conditions of excessive calcium needs, such as during the egg-laying cycle of birds. Knowing the functional form of vitamin D in the target organs has facilitated an investigation into the molecular mechanism of action. This has given rise to the idea that the active form of vitamin D, namely, 1,25-$(OH)_2D_3$, functions in the target organs by binding to a specific receptor cytosol protein and that it is then transferred to the nucleus where it facilitates transcription of genetic information coding for calcium and phosphorus transport proteins. The nature of these proteins remains unknown, and the detailed mechanism of the calcium and phosphorus transfer reactions remains to be elucidated. The interaction between vitamin D and other well-established endocrine systems is now becoming elucidated, which will provide important new insights into metabolic bone disease and diseases of calcium and phosphorus homeostasis.

Finally the discovery and chemical synthesis of the vitamin D metabolites and their analogs have provided important new tools to the medical world for the treatment of metabolic bone diesease. Such diseases as hypoparathyroidism, renal osteodystrophy, corticoid-induced osteoporosis, and certain types of vitamin D-resistant rickets appear to be well on their way toward medical management. Other possible disease states are under investigation for possible application of the vitamin D metabolites. The vitamin D metabolites, therefore, represent an important new contribution of basic science to the practice of medicine.

References

Adams, T. H., Norman, A. W.: Studies on the mechanism of action of calciferol. I. Basic parameters of vitamin D-mediated calcium transport. J. Biol. Chem. *245*, 4421–4431 (1970)

Adams, T. H., Wong, R. G., Norman, A. W.: Studies on the mechanism of action of calciferol. II. Effects of the polyene antibiotic, filipin, on vitamin D-mediated calcium transport. J. Biol. Chem. *245*, 4432–4442 (1970)

Albright, F., Bloomberg, E., Drake, T., Sulkowitch, H.: A comparison of the effects of A.T. 10 (dihydrotachysterol) and vitamin D on calcium and phosphorus metabolism in hypoparathyroidism. J. Clin. Invest. *17*, 317–329 (1938)

Anderson, H. C.: Vesicles associated with calcification in the matrix of epiphyseal cartilage. J. Cell Biol. *41*, 59–72 (1969)

Anderson, H. C.: Matrix vesicle calcification. Fed. Proc. *35*, 105–108 (1976)

Anderson, H. C., Sajdera, S. W.: Calcification of rachitic cartilage to study matrix vesicle function. Fed. Proc. *35*, 148–153 (1976)

Arnaud, S. B., Stickler, G. B., Haworth, J. C.: Serum 25-hydroxy-vitamin D in infantile rickets. Pediatrics *57*, 221–225 (1976)

Arnaud, S. B., Matthusen, M., Gilkinson, J. B., Goldsmith, R. S.: Components of 25-hydroxyvitamin D in serum of young children in upper mid-western United States. Am. J. Clin. Nutr. *30*, 1082–1086 (1977)

Arnold, B. M., Kuttner, M., Willis, D. M., Hitchman, A. J. W., Harrison, J. E., Murray, T. M.: Radioimmunoassay studies of intestinal calcium-binding protein in the pig. II. The distribution of intestinal CaBP in pig tissue. Can. J. Physiol. Pharmacol. *53*, 1135–1140 (1975)

Askew, F. A., Bourdillon, R. B., Bruce, H. M., Jenkins, R. G. C., Webster, T. A.: The distillation of vitamin D. Proc. R. Soc. Lond. [Biol.] *107*, 76–90 (1931)

Avioli, L. V., Lee, S. W., McDonald, J. E., Lund, J., DeLuca, H. F.: Metabolism of vitamin D_3-^3H in human subjects: distribution in blood, bile, feces, and urine. J. Clin. Invest. *46*, 983–992 (1967).

Baelen, H. van, Bouillon, R., DeMoor, P.: Binding of 25-hydroxycholecalciferol in tissues. J. Biol. Chem. *252*, 2515–2518 (1977)

Baksi, S. N., Kenny, A. D.: Vitamin D_3 metabolism in immature Japanese quail: effects of ovarian hormones. Endocrinology *101*, 1216–1220 (1977)

Balsan, S., Garabedian, M., Pezant, E., Sorgniard, R., Holick, M. F., DeLuca, H. F.: Biologic and therapeutic effects of 1α-hydroxyvitamin D in children. In: Calcium regulating hormones. Talmage, R. V., Owen, M., Parsons, J. A. (eds.), pp. 439–447. Excerpta Medica 1975

Bar, A., Wasserman, R. H.: Control of calcium absorption and intestinal calcium-binding protein synthesis. Biochem. Biophys. Res. Commun. *54*, 191–196 (1973)

Barnes, M. J., Constable, B. J., Morton, L. F., Kodicek, E.: Bone collagen metabolism in vitamin D deficiency. Biochem. J. *132*, 113–115 (1973)

Bauer, G. C. H., Carlsson, A., Lindquist, B.: Evaluation of accretion, resorption, and exchange reactions in the skeleton. Kungl. Fysiograf. Sallskapets I Lund Forhandlingar *25*, 3–18 (1955)

Baxter, L. A., DeLuca, H. F.: Stimulation of 25-hydroxyvitamin D_3-1α-hydroxylase by phosphate depletion. J. Biol. Chem. *251*, 3158–3161 (1976)

Baxter, L. A., DeLuca, H. F., Bonjour, J.-P., Fleisch, H.: Inhibition of vitamin D metabolism by ethane-1-hydroxy-1,1-diphosphonate. Arch. Biochem. Biophys. *164*, 655–662 (1974)

Bayard, F., Bec, Ph., That, H. T., Louvet, J. P.: Plasma 25-hydroxy-cholecalciferol in chronic renal failure. Europ. J. Clin. Invest. *3*, 447–450 (1973)

Bell, D. J., Freeman, B. M. (eds.): Physiology and biochemistry of the domestic fowl. London: Academic Press 1971, Vol. 3

Bhattacharyya, M. H., DeLuca, H. F.: The regulation of rat liver calciferol-25-hydroxylase. J. Biol. Chem. *248*, 2969–2973 (1973)

Bhattacharyya, M. H., DeLuca, H. F.: The regulation of calciferol-25-hydroxylase in the chick. Biochem. Biophys. Res. Commun. *59*, 734–741 (1974a)

Bhattacharyya, M. H., DeLuca, H. F.: Subcellular location of rat liver calciferol-25-hydroxylase. Arch. Biochem. Biophys. *160*, 58–62 (1974b)

Bikle, D. D., Rasmussen, H.: The ionic control of 1,25-dihydroxyvitamin D_3 production in isolated chick renal tubules. J. Clin. Invest. *55*, 292–298 (1975)

Bikle, D. D., Murphy, E. W., Rasmussen, H.: The ionic control of 1,25-dihydroxyvitamin D_3 synthesis in isolated chick renal mitochondria. J. Clin. Invest. *55*, 299–304 (1975)

Birge, S. J., Haddad, J. G.: 25-Hydroxycholecalciferol stimulation of muscle metabolism. J. Clin. Invest. *56*, 1100–1107 (1975)

Bloch, K.: The biological synthesis of cholesterol. Science *150*, 19–22 (1965)

Blumberg, A., Aebi, H., Hurni, H., Schönholzer, G.: Das Verteilungsmuster von C^{14}-ergocalciferol (vitamin D_2) bei der Ratte und beim Rhesusaffen. Helv. Physiol. Acta *18*, 56–71 (1960)

Blunt, J. W., DeLuca, H. F.: The synthesis of 25-hydroxycholecalciferol. A biologically active metabolite of vitamin D_3. Biochemistry *8*, 671–675 (1969)

Blunt, J. W. Tanaka, Y., DeLuca, H. F.: The biological activity of 25-hydroxycholecalciferol, a metabolite of vitamin D_3. Proc. Natl. Acad. Sci. USA *61*, 1503–1506 (1968a)

Blunt, J. W., DeLuca, H. F., Schnoes, H. K.: 25-Hydroxycholecalciferol. A biologically active metabolite of vitamin D_3. Biochemistry *7*, 3317–3322 (1968b)

Bonjour, J.-P., Fleisch, H.: The effect of vitamin D and its metabolites on the renal handling of phosphate. In: Vitamin D: biochemical, chemical and clinical aspects related to calcium metabolism. Norman, A. W., Schaefer, K., Coburn, J. W., DeLuca, H. F., Fraser, D., Grigoleit, H. G., von Herrath, D. (eds.), pp. 419–431. Berlin: de Gruyter 1977

Bonjour, J.-P., Preston, C., Fleisch, H.: Role of 1,25-dihydroxyvitamin D_3 in renal handling of inorganic phosphate in rats — Abstr. Experientia *33*, 777 (1977)

Bonjour, J.-P., Russell, R. G. G., Morgan, D. B., Fleisch, H. A.: Relationship between calcium accretion rate into bone and intestinal calcium absorption in diphosphonate treated rats — Abstr. Europ. J. Clin. Invest. *2*, 274 (1972)

Bonjour, J.-P., DeLuca, H. F., Fleisch, H., Trechsel, U., Matejowec, L. A., Omdahl, J. L.: Reversal of the EHDP inhibition of calcium absorption by 1,25-dihydroxycholecalciferol. Europ. J. Clin. Invest. *3*, 44–48 (1973)

Bonjour, J.-P., Trechsel, U., Fleisch, H., Schenk, R., DeLuca, H. F., Baxter, L. A.: Action of 1,25-dihydroxyvitamin D_3 and a diphosphonate on calcium metabolism in rats. Am. J. Physiol. *229*, 402–408 (1975)

Bonjour, J.-P., Trechsel, U., Trohler, U., Fleisch, H., Baxter, L. A., DeLuca, H. F.: Influence of a diphosphonate and 1,25-dihydroxycholecalciferol on calcium metabolism. In: Calcium metabolism, bone and metabolic bone diseases. Kuhlencordt, F., Kruse, H.-P. (eds.), pp. 251–255. Berlin, Heidelberg, New York: Springer 1976

Booth, B. E., Tsai, H. C., Morris, C.: Parathyroidectomy reduces 25-hydroxyvitamin D_3-1α-hydroxylase activity in hypocalcemic vitamin D-deficient chick. J. Clin. Invest. *60*, 1314–1320 (1977)

Bordier, P., Miravet, L., Tun Chot, S., Hioco, D.: Evidences of a direct effect of vitamin D_3 or 25-hydroxycholecalciferol upon human adult bone mineralization. In: Cellular mechanisms for calcium transfer and homeostasis. Nichols, G. (Jr.), Wasserman, R. H. (eds.). pp. 459–460. New York: Academic Press 1971

Bordier, P., Ryckwaert, A., Marie, P., Miravet, L., Norman, A., Rasmussen, H.: Vitamin D metabolites and bone mineralization in man. In: Vitamin D: biochemical, chemical and clinical aspects related to calcium metabolism. Norman, A. W., Schaefer, K., Coburn, J. W., DeLuca, H. F., Fraser, D., Grigoleit, H. G., von Herrath, D. (eds.). pp. 897–911. Berlin: de Gruyter 1977

Boris, A., Hurley, J. F., Trmal, T.: Relative activities of some metabolites and analogs of cholecalciferol in stimulation of tibia ash weight in chicks otherwise deprived of vitamin D. J. Nutr. *107*, 194–198 (1977)

Botham, K. M., Ghazarian, J. G., Kream, B. E., DeLuca, H. F.: Isolation of a potent inhibitor of 25-hydroxyvitamin D_3-1-hydroxylase from rat serum. Biochemistry *15*, 2130–2135 (1976)

Bouillon, R., Van Baelen, H., Rombauts, W., DeMoor, P.: The purification and characterisation of the human-serum binding protein for the 25-hydroxycholecalciferol (transcalciferin). Identity with group-specific component. Europ. J. Biochem. *66*, 285–291 (1976)

Boyle, I. T. Gray, R. W., DeLuca, H. F.: Regulation by calcium of in vivo synthesis of 1,25-dihydroxycholecalciferol and 21,25-dihydroxycholecalciferol. Proc. Natl. Acad. Sci. USA *68*, 2131–2134 (1971)

Boyle, I. T., Miravet, L., Gray, R. W., Holick, M. F., DeLuca, H. F.: The response of intestinal calcium transport to 25-hydroxy and 1,25-dihydroxy vitamin D in nephrectomized rats. Endocrinology *90*, 605–608 (1972a)

Boyle, I. T., Gray, R. W., Omdahl, J. L., DeLuca, H. F.: Calcium control of the in vivo biosynthesis of 1,25-dihydroxyvitamin D_3: Nicolaysen's endogenous factor. In: Endocrinology 1971. Taylor, S. (ed.). pp. 468–476. Heinemann Medical Books 1972b

Boyle, I. T., Omdahl, J. L., Gray, R. W., DeLuca, H. F.: The biological activity and metabolism of 24,25-dihydroxyvitamin D_3. J. Biol. Chem. *248*, 4174–4180 (1973)

Bricker, N. S., Slatopolsky, E., Reiss, E., Avioli, L. V.: Calcium, phosphorus and bone in renal disease and transplantation. Arch. Internal Med. *123*, 543–553 (1969)

Brickman, A. S., Coburn, J. W., Norman, A. W.: Action of 1,25-dihydroxycholecalciferol, a potent, kidney-produced metabolite of vitamin D_3, in uremic man. New Engl. J. Med. *287*, 891–895 (1972)

Brickman, A., Coburn, J. W., Kurakawa, K., Bethune, J. E., Harrison, H. E., Norman, A. W.: Actions of 1,25-dihydroxyvitamin D_3 in patients with hypophosphatemic vitamin D-resistant rickets. New Engl. J. Med. *289*, 495–498 (1973)

Brickman, A. S., Sherrard, D. J., Jowsey, J., Singer, F. R., Baylink, D. J., Maloney, N., Massry, S. G., Norman, A. W., Coburn, J. W.: 1,25-Dihydroxycholecalciferol. Effect on skeletal lesions and plasma parathyroid hormone levels in uremic osteodystrophy. Arch. Intern. Med. *134*, 883–888 (1974)

Brumbaugh, P. F., Haussler, M. R.: Nuclear and cytoplasmic receptors for 1,25-dihydroxycholecalciferol in intestinal mucosa. Biochem. Biophys. Res. Commun. *51*, 74–80 (1973)

Brumbaugh, P. F., Haussler, M. R.: 1α,25-Dihydroxycholecalciferol receptors in intestine. I. Association of 1α,25-dihydroxycholecalciferol with intestinal mucosa chromatin. J. Biol. Chem. *249*, 1251–1257 (1974a)

Brumbaugh, P. F., Haussler, M. R.: 1α,25-Dihydroxycholecalciferol receptors in intestine. II. Temperature-dependent transfer of the hormone to chromatin via a specific cytosol receptor. J. Biol. Chem. *249*, 1258–1262 (1974b)

Brumbaugh, P. F., Hughes, M. R., Haussler, M. R.: Cytoplasmic and nuclear binding components for 1α,25-dihydroxyvitamin D_3 in chick parathyroid glands. Proc. Natl. Acad. Sci. USA *72*, 4871–4875 (1975)

Bruns, E. H., Avioli, L. V.: The activity and the synthesis of CaBP during vitamin D replacement in the rachitic rat. In: Calcium regulating hormones. Talmage, R. V., Owen, M., Parsons, J. A. (eds.). pp. 336–445. Amsterdam: Excerpta Medica 1975

Bruns, M. E. H., Fliesher, E. B., Avioli, L. V.: Control of vitamin D-dependent calcium binding protein in rat intestine by growth and fasting. J. Biol. Chem. *252*, 4145–4150 (1977)

Canfield, R., Rosner, W., Skinner, J., McWhorter, J., Resnick, L., Feldman, F., Kammerman, S., Ryan, K., Kunigonis, M., Bohne, W.: Diphosphonate therapy of Pagets disease of bone. J. Clin. Endocrinol. Metab. *44*, 96–106 (1977)

Carlsson, A.: Tracer experiments on the effect of vitamin D on the skeletal metabolism of calcium and phosphorus. Acta Physiol. Scand *26*, 212–220 (1952)

Carlsson, A.: Experiments with radiocalcium on the interrelationships between vitamin D and dietary calcium and phosphorus. Acta Pharmacol. Toxicol. *9*, 32–40 (1953)

Carré, M., Ayigbede, O., Miravet, L., Rasmussen, H.: The effect of prednisolone upon the metabolism and action of 25-hydroxy and 1,25-dihydroxyvitamin D_3. Proc. Natl. Acad. Sci. USA *71*, 2996–3000 (1974)

Castillo, L., Tanaka, Y., DeLuca, H. F., Sunde, M. L.: The stimulation of 25-hydroxyvitamin D_3-1α-hydroxylase by estrogen. Arch. Biochem. Biophys. *179*, 211–217 (1977)

Castillo, L., Tanaka, Y., DeLuca, H. F., Ikekawa, N.: On the physiological role of 1,24,25-trihydroxyvitamin D_3. Mineral Electrolyte Metab. *7*, 198–207 (1978)

Chan, J. C. M., DeLuca, H. F.: Growth velocity in a child on prolonged hemodialysis. Beneficial effect of 1α-hydroxyvitamin D_3. J. Am. Med. Assoc. *238*, 2053–2054 (1977)

Chan, J. C. M., Oldham, S. B., Holick, M. F., DeLuca, H. F.: 1α-Hydroxy-vitamin D_3 in chronic renal failure. A potent analogue of the kidney hormone, 1,25-dihydroxycholecalciferol. J. Am. Med. Assoc. *234*, 47–52 (1975)

Chan, J. C. M., Oldham, S. B., DeLuca, H. F.: Effectiveness of 1α-hydroxyvitamin D in children with renal osteodystophy associated with hemodialysis. J. Pediat. *90*, 820–824 (1977)

Chen, P. S. (Jr.), Bosmann, H. B.: Effect of vitamin D_2 and D_3 in serum calcium and phosphorus in rachitic chicks. J. Nutr. *83*, 133–139 (1964)

Chen, T. C., DeLuca, H. F.: Stimulation of [^{3}H] uridine incorporation into nuclear RNA of rat kidney by vitamin D metabolites. Arch. Biochem. Biophys. *156*, 321–327 (1973)

Chen, T. C., Weber, J. C., DeLuca, H. F.: On the subcellular location of vitamin D metabolites in intestine. J. Biol. Chem. *245*, 3776–3780 (1970)

Chen, T. C., Castillo, L., Korycka-Dahl, M., DeLuca, H. F.: Role of vitamin D metabolites in phosphate transport of rat intestine. J. Nutr. *104*, 1056–1060 (1974)

Chertow, B. S., Baylink, D. J., Wergedal, J. E., Su, M. H. H., Norman, A. W.: Decrease in serum immunoreactive parathyroid hormone in rats and in parathyroid hormone secretion in vitro by 1,25-dihydroxycholecalciferol. J. Clin. Invest. *56*, 668–678 (1975)

Chesney, R. W., Moorthy, A. V., Eisman, J. A., Jax, D. K., Mazess, R. B., DeLuca, H. F.: Increased growth after long-term oral 1α,25-dihydroxyvitamin D_3 in childhood renal osteodystrophy. New Engl. J. Med. *298*, 238–242 (1978)

Chick, H., Dalzell, E. J., Hume, E. M.: Studies of rickets in Vienna 1919–1922. Medical Research Council Special Report No. 77 (1923)

Cinti, D. L., Golub, E. E., Bronner, F.: 25-Hydroxycholecalciferol: high affinity substrate for hepatic cytochrome P-450. Biochem. Biophys. Res. Commun. *72*, 546–553 (1976)

Colston, K. W., Evans, I. M. A., Galante, L., MacIntyre, I., Moss, D. W.: Regulation of vitamin D metabolism: factors influencing the rate of formation of 1,25-dihydroxycholecalciferol by kidney homogenates. Biochem. J. *134*, 817–820 (1973)

Corradino, R. A., Wasserman, R. H.: Strontium inhibition of vitamin D_3-induced calcium-binding protein (CaBP) and calcium absorption in chick intestine. Proc. Soc. Exp. Biol. Med. *133*, 960–963 (1970)

Corradino, R. A., Ebel, J. G., Craig, P. H., Taylor, A. N., Wasserman, R. H.: Calcium absorption and the vitamin D_3-dependent calcium-binding protein. I. Inhibition by dietary strontium. Calc. Tissue Res. 7, 81–92 (1971a)

Corradino, R. A., Ebel, J. G., Craig, P. H., Taylor, A. N., Wasserman, R. H.: Calcium absorption and the vitamin D_3-dependent calcium-binding protein. II. Recovery from dietary strontium inhibition. Calc. Tissue Res. *7*, 93–102 (1971b)

Daiger, S. P., Schanfield, M. S., Cavalli-Sforza, L. L.: Group-specific component (Gc) proteins bind vitamin D and 25-hydroxyvitamin D. Proc. Natl. Acad. Sci. USA *72*, 2076–2080 (1975)

Daniels, F., Jr.: Man and radiant energy: solar radiation. In: Handbook of Physiology. Sect. 4; Adaptation to environment. Field, F. (Jr.) (ed.). pp. 969–987. Baltimore: Williams and Wilkins 1964

Davie, M. W. J., Chalmers, T. M., Hunter, J. O., Pelc, B., Kodicek, E.: 1α-Hydroxycholecalciferol in chronic renal failure. Ann. Intern. Med. *84*, 281–285 (1976)

Deftos, L. J.: Calcitonin: hormonal and regulatory mechanisms. In: Proceedings of the sixth parathyroid conference, University of British Columbia, Vancouver, Canada — Abstract 1977, p. 133

DeLuca, H. F.: Mechanism of action and metabolic fate of vitamin D. Vitam. Horm. *25*, 315–367 (1967)

DeLuca, H. F.: Metabolism and function of vitamin D. In: The fat-soluble vitamins. DeLuca, H. F., Suttie, J. W. (eds.). pp. 3–20. Madison: University Press 1970

DeLuca, H. F.: Minireview: regulation of vitamin D metabolism. Life Sci. *17*, 1351–1358 (1975)

DeLuca, H. F.: Vitamin D. In: The fat-soluble vitamins. Vol. 2: Handbook of lipid research. DeLuca, H. F. (ed.). pp. 69–132. New York: Plenum Press 1978

DeLuca, H. F., Avioli, L. V.: Renal osteodystrophy. In: Renal Disease. 4th ed. Black, D. (ed.). Oxford: Blackwell Scientific 1978 (in press)

DeLuca, H. F., Weller, M., Blunt, J. W., Neville, P. F.: Synthesis, biological activity, and metabolism of 22,23-^{3}H-vitamin D_4. Arch. Biochem. Biophys. *124*, 122–128 (1968)

DeLuca, H. F., Blunt, J. W., Rikkers, H.: VII. Vitamin D Biogenesis. In: The vitamins. Sebrell, W. H. (Jr.), Harris, R. S. (eds.). pp. 213–230. New York: Academic Press 1971

Dowdle, E. B., Schachter, D., Schenker, H.: Requirement for vitamin D for the active transport of calcium by the intestine. Am. J. Physiol. *198*, 269–274 (1960)

Drescher, D., DeLuca, H. F.: Vitamin D stimulated calcium binding protein from rat intestinal mucosa. Purification and some properties. Biochemistry *10*, 2302–2307 (1971a)

Drescher, D., DeLuca, H. F.: Possible precursor of vitamin D stimulated calcium binding protein in rats. Biochemistry *10*, 2308–2312 (1971b)

Drezner, M. K., Neelon, F. A., Haussler, M., McPherson, H. T., Lebovitz, H. E.: 1,25-Dihydroxycholecalciferol deficiency: the probable cause of hypocalcemia and metabolic bone disease in pseudohypoparathyroidism. J. Clin. Endocrinol. Metab. *42*, 621–628 (1976)

Ebel, J. G., Taylor, A. N., Wasserman, R. H.: Vitamin D induced calcium binding protein of intestinal mucosa in relation to vitamin D dose level and lag period. Am. J. Clin. Nutr. *22*, 431–436 (1969)

Eicher, E. M., Southard, J. L., Scriver, C. R., Glorieux, F. H.: Hypophosphatemia: mouse model for human familial hypophosphatemic (vitamin D-resistant) rickets. Proc. Natl. Acad. Sci. USA *73*, 4667–4671 (1976)

Eichmann, C.: Eine beriberi-ähnliche Krankheit der Hühner. Virchows Arch. Pathol. Anat. Physiol. *148*, 523–532 (1897)

Eisman, J. A., DeLuca, H. F.: Intestinal 1,25-dihydroxyvitamin D_3 binding protein: specificity of binding. Steroids *30*, 245–257 (1977)

Eisman, J. A., Hamstra, A. J., Kream, B. E., DeLuca, H. F.: 1,25-Dihydroxyvitamin D in biological fluids: a simplified and sensitive assay. Science *193*, 1021–1023 (1976a)

Eisman, J. A., Hamstra, A. J., Kream, B. E., DeLuca, H. F.: A sensitive, precise and convenient method for determination of 1,25-dihydroxy-vitamin D in human plasma. Arch. Biochem. Biophys. *176*, 235–243 (1976b)

Eisman, J. A., Shepard, R. M., DeLuca, H. F.: Determination of 25-hydroxyvitamin D_2 and 25-hydroxyvitamin D_3 in human plasma using high-pressure liquid chromatography. Anal. Biochem. *80*, 298–305 (1977)

Ellis, G., Woodhead, J. S., Cooke, W. T.: Serum 25-hydroxyvitamin D concentrations in adolescent boys. Lancet *1*, 825–828 (1977)

Esvelt, R. P., DeLuca, H. F., Schnoes, H. K.: Vitamin D_3 from rat skins irradiated in vitro with ultraviolet light. Arch. Biochem. Biophys. *188*, 282–286 (1978)

Favus, M. J., Kimberg, D. V., Millar, G. N., Gershon, E.: Effects of cortisone administration on the metabolism and localization of 25-hydroxycholecalciferol in the rat. J. Clin. Invest. *52*, 1328–1335 (1973b)

Favus, M. J., Walling, M. W., Kimberg, D. V.: Effects of 1,25-dihydroxycholecalciferol on intestinal calcium transport in cortisone-treated rats. J. Clin. Invest. *52*, 1680–1685 (1973b)

Favus, M. J., Walling, M. W., Kimberg, D. V: Effects of dietary calcium restriction and chronic thyroparathyroidectomy on the metabolism of [^{3}H]-25-hydroxyvitamin D_3 and the active transport of calcium by rat intestine. J. Clin. Invest. *53*, 1139–1148 (1974)

Fleisch, H., Russell, R. G. G., Bisaz, S., Casey, P. A., Mühlbauer, R. C.: The influence of pyrophosphate analogues (diphosphonates) on the precipitation and dissolution of calcium phosphate in vitro and in vivo. Calc. Tissue Res. *2* Suppl., 10–10A (1968)

Forte, L. R., Nickols, G. A., Anast, C. S.: Renal adenylate cyclase and the interrelationship between parathyroid hormone and vitamin D in the regulation of urinary phosphate and adenosine cyclic 3',5'-monophosphate excretion. J. Clin. Invest. *57*, 559–568 (1976)

Fournier, A. E., Bordier, P. J., Gueris, J., Chanard, J., Marie, P., Ferriere, C., Osario, M., Bedrossian, J., DeLuca, H. F.: 1α-Hydroxy-cholecalciferol and 25-hydroxycholecalciferol in renal bone disease. In: Calcified tissues 1975. Pors Nielsen, S., Hjørting-Hansen, E. (eds.). pp. 226–235. Copenhagen: FADL's Forlag 1976

Fraser, D. R., Kodicek, E.: Unique biosynthesis by kidney of a biologically active vitamin D metabolite. Nature *228*, 764–766 (1970)

Fraser, D. R., Kodicek, E.: Regulation of 25-hydroxycholecalciferol-1-hydroxylase activity in kidney by parathyroid hormone. Nature New Biol. *241*, 163–166 (1973)

Fraser, D., Kooh, S. W., Kind, H. P., Holick, M. F., Tanaka, Y., DeLuca, H. F.: Pathogenesis of hereditary vitamin D dependent rickets: an inborn error of vitamin D metabolism involving defective conversion of 25-hydroxyvitamin D to 1α,25-dihydroxyvitamin D. New Engl. J. Med. *289*, 817–822 (1973)

Frost, H. M.: Bone dynamics in osteoporosis and osteomalacia. Henry Ford Hospital Surgical Monograph Series. Springfield: Charles A. Thomas 1966

Fullmer, C. S., Wasserman, R. H.: Bovine intestinal calcium-binding proteins. Purification and some properties. Biochim. Biophys. Acta *317*, 172–186 (1973)

Funk, C.: On the chemical nature of the substance which cures polyneuritis in birds induced by a diet of polished rice. J. Physiol. *43*, 395–400 (1911)

Galante, L., MacAuley, S. J., Colston, K. .W., MacIntyre, I.: Effect of parathyroid extract on vitamin D metabolism. Lancet *1*, 985–988 (1972a)

Galante, L., Colston, K. W., MacAuley, S. J., MacIntyre, I.: Effect of calcitonin on vitamin D metabolism. Nature *238*, 271–273 (1972b)

Galante, L., Colston, K. W., Evans, I. M. A., Byfield, P. G. H., Matthews, E. W., MacIntyre, I.: The regulation of vitamin D metabolism. Nature *244*, 438–440 (1973)

Garabedian, M., Holick, M. F., DeLuca, H. F., Boyle, I. T.: Control of 25-hydroxycholecalciferol metabolism by the parathyroid glands. Proc. Natl. Acad. Sci. USA *69*, 1673–1676 (1972)

Garabedian, M., Tanaka, Y., Holick, M. F., DeLuca, H. F.: Response of intestinal calcium transport and bone calcium mobilization to 1,25-dihydroxyvitamin D_3 in thyroparathyroidectomized rats. Endocrinology *94*, 1022–1027 (1974)

Garabedian, M., Corvol, M. T., Baily du Bois, M., Lieberherr, M., Balsan, S.: The biological activity of 24,25-dihydroxycholecalciferol on cultured chondrocytes and its in vitro production in cartilage and calvarium. In: Proceedings of the sixth parathyroid conference. University of British Columbia, Vancouver, Canada. Abstract (1977), p. 160

Ghazarian, J. G., DeLuca, H. F.: 25-Hydroxycholecalciferol-1-hydroxylase: a specific requirement for NADPH and a hemoprotein component in chick kidney mitochondria. Arch. Biochem. Biophys. *160*, 63–72 (1974)

Ghazarian, J. G., Schnoes, H. K., DeLuca, H. F.: Mechanism of 25-hydroxycholecalciferol 1α-hydroxylation. Incorporation of oxygen-18 into the 1α position of 25-hydroxycholecalciferol. Biochemistry *12*, 2555–2558 (1973)

Ghazarian, J. G., Jefcoate, C. R., Knutson, J. C., Orme-Johnson, W. H., DeLuca, H. F.: Mitochondrial cytochrome P_{450}: a component of chick kidney 25-hydroxycholecalciferol-1α-hydroxylase. J. Biol. Chem. *249*, 3026–3033 (1974)

Ghazarian, J. G., Hsu, P.-Y., Peterson, B. L.: Chick kidney microsomal cytochrome P-450 involvement in the metabolism of 25-hydroxy-vitamin D_3. Arch. Biochem. Biophys. *184*, 596–604 (1977)

Glimcher, M. J.: Macromolecular aggregation stage and reactivity of collagen in calcification. Soc. Gen. Physiol. *6*, 53–84 (1959)

Glorieux, F., Scriver, C. R.: Loss of a parathyroid-sensitive component of phosphate transport in X-linked hypophosphatemia. Science *175*, 997–1000 (1972)

Glorieux, F. H., Scriver, C. R., Reade, T. M., Goldman, H., Roseborough, A.: Use of phosphate and vitamin D to prevent dwarfism and rickets in X-linked hypophosphatemia. New Engl. J. Med. *287*, 481–487 (1972)

Glorieux, F. H., Scriver, C. R., Holick, M. F., DeLuca, H. F.: X-linked hypophosphatemic rickets: inadequate therapeutic response to 1,25-dihydroxycholecalciferol. Lancet *2*, 287–289 (1973)

Goldblatt, H., Soames, K. M.: Studies on the fat soluble growth-promoting factor (I) storage (II) synthesis. Biochem. J. *17*, 446–453 (1923)

Gonnerman, W. A., Toverud, S. U., Ramp, W. K., Mechanic, G. L.: Effects of dietary vitamin D and calcium on lysyl oxidase activity in chick bone metaphyses. Proc. Soc. Exp. Biol. Med. *151*, 453–456 (1976)

Goodman, D. B. P., Haussler, M. R., Rasmussen, H.: Vitamin D_3 induced alteration of microvillar membrane lipid composition. Biochem. Biophys. Res. Commun. *46*, 80–86 (1972)

Gran, F. C.: The retention of parenterally injected calcium in rachitic dogs. Acta Physiol. Scand. *50*, 132–139 (1960)

Gray, R., Boyle, I., DeLuca, H. F.: Vitamin D metabolism: the role of kidney tissue. Science *172*, 1232–1234 (1971)

Gray, R. W., Omdahl, J. L., Ghazarian, J. G., DeLuca, H. F.: 25-Hydroxy-cholecalcificerol-1-hydroxylase: subcellular location and properties. J. Biol. Chem. *247*, 7528–7532 (1972)

Greaves, J. D., Schmidt, C. L. A.: The role played by bile in the absorption of vitamin D in the rat. J. Biol. Chem. *102*, 101–112 (1933)

Grijns, G.: Researches on vitamins 1900–1911. J. Nooduijnen zoon Gorinchem, 1935. As cited in: Sebrell, W. H., Harris, R. S. (eds.): The vitamins. p. 99. New York: Academic Press 1972, Vol. 5

Haddad, J. G., Birge, S. J.: Widespread, specific binding of 25-hydroxycholecalciferol in rat tissues. J. Biol. Chem. *250*, 299–303 (1975)

Haddad, J. G., Stamp, T. C. B.: Circulating 25-hydroxyvitamin D in man. Am. J. Med. *57*, 57–62 (1974)

Haddad, J. G., Walgate, J.: 25-Hydroxyvitamin D transport in human plasma. J. Biol. Chem. *251*, 4803–4809 (1976)

Haddad, J. G., Chyu, K. J., Hahn, T. J., Stamp, T. C. B.: Serum concentrations of 25-hydroxyvitamin D in sex-linked hypophosphatemic vitamin D-resistant rickets. J. Lab. Clin. Med. *81*, 22–27 (1973a)

Haddad, J. G., Hahn, T. J., Birge, S. F.: Vitamin D metabolites specific binding by rat intestinal cytosol. Biochim. Biophys. Acta *329*, 93–97 (1973b)

Haddad, J. G., Walgate, J., Min, C., Hahn, T.: Vitamin D metabolite-binding proteins in human tissue. Biochim. Biophys. Acta *444*, 921–925 (1976)

Hahn, T. J., Avioli, L. V.: Hepatic bioactivation of vitamin D and clinical implications. In: Vitamin D: biochemical, chemical and clinical aspects related to calcium metabolism. Norman, A. W., Schaefer, K., Coburn, J. W., DeLuca, H. F., Fraser, D., Grigoleit, H. G., Herrath, D. von (eds.). pp. 737–745. Berlin: de Gruyter 1977

Hahn, T. J., Hendin, B. A., Scharp, C. R., Haddad, J. G.: Effect of chronic anticonvulsant therapy on serum 25-hydroxycalciferol levels in adults. New Engl. J. Med. *287*, 900–904 (1972)

Hallick, R. B., DeLuca, H. F.: Vitamin D_3-stimulated template activity of chromatin from rat intestine. Proc. Natl. Acad. Sci. USA *63*, 528–531 (1969)

Hallick, R. B., DeLuca, H. F.: 25-Hydroxydihydrotachysterol$_3$ – biosynthesis in vivo and in vitro. J. Biol. Chem. *246*, 5733–5738 (1971)

Hallick, R. B., DeLuca, H. F.: Metabolites of dihydrotachysterol$_3$ in target tissues. J. Biol. Chem. *247*, 91–97 (1972)

Harmeyer, J., DeLuca, H. F.: Calcium-binding protein and calcium absorption after vitamin D administration. Arch. Biochem. Biophys. *133*, 247–254 (1969)

Harrison, H. E., Harrison, H. C.: The renal excretion of inorganic phosphate in relation to the action of vitamin D and parathyroid hormone. J. Clin. Invest. *20*, 47–55 (1941)

Harrison, H. E., Harrison, H. C.: Transfer of Ca^{45} across intestinal wall in vitro in relation to action of vitamin D and cortisol. Am. J. Physiol. *199*, 265–271 (1960)

Harrison, H. E., Harrison, H. C.: Intestinal transport of phosphate: action of vitamin D, calcium, and potassium. Am. J. Physiol. *201*, 1007–1012 (1961)

Harrison, H. E., Harrison, H. C.: Sodium, potassium, and intestinal transport of glucose, 1-tyrosine, phosphate, and calcium. Am. J. Physiol. *205*, 107–111 (1963)

Harrison, H. E., Harrison, H. C.: Vitamin D and permeability of intestinal mucosa to calcium. Am. J. Physiol. *208*, 370–374 (1965)

Harrison, H. C., Harrison, H. E.: Calcium transport by rat colon in vitro. Am. J. Physiol. *217*, 121–125 (1969)

Harrison, H. C., Harrison, H. E.: Comparison of activity of 25-hydroxy-cholecalciferol and dihydrotachysterol$_2$ in the thyroparathyroidectomized rat. Proc. Soc. Exp. Biol. Med. *136*, 411–414 (1971)

Harrison, H. C., Harrison, H. E., Park, E. A.: Vitamin D and citrate metabolism. Effect of vitamin D in rats fed diets adequate in both calcium and phosphorus. Am. J. Physiol. *192*, 432–436 (1958)

Hart, E. B., McCollum, E. V., Steenbock, H., Humphrey, G. C.: Physiological effect on growth and reproduction of rations balanced from restricted sources. Wis. Expt. Station Bull. *17*, 131–205 (June 1911)

Haussler, M. R., Norman, A. W.: The subcellular distribution of physiological doses of vitamin D_3. Arch. Biochem. Biophys. *118*, 145–153 (1967)

Haussler, M. R., Myrtle, J. F., Norman, A. W.: The association of a metabolite of vitamin D_3 with intestinal mucosa chromatin in vivo. J. Biol. Chem. *243*, 4055–4064 (1968)

Haussler, M. R., Zerwekh, J. E., Hesse, R. H., Rizzardo, E., Pechet, M. M.: Biological activity of 1α-hydroxycholecalciferol, a synthetic analog of the hormonal form of vitamin D_3. Proc. Natl. Acad. Sci. USA *70*, 2248–2252 (1973)

Haussler, M. R., Baylink, D. J., Hughes, M. R., Brumbaugh, P. F., Wergedal, J. E., Shen, F. H., Nielsen, R. L., Counts, S. J., Bursac, K. M., McCain, T. A.: The assay of 1α,25-dihydroxyvitamin D_3: physiologic and pathologic modulation of circulating hormone levels. Clin. Endocrinol. *5*, 151s–165s (1976)

Haussler, M., Hughes, M., Baylink, D., Littledike, E. T., Cork, D., Pitt, M.: Influence of phosphate depletion on the biosynthesis and circulating level of 1α,25-dihydroxyvitamin D. In: Phosphate metabolism. Massry, S. G., Ritz, E. (eds.). pp. 233–250. New York: Plenum Press 1977

Havinga, E.: Vitamin D, example and challenge. Experientia *29*, 1181–1316 (1973)

Heaney, R. P.: Vitamin D and osteoporosis. In: Vitamin D: biochemical, chemical and clinical aspects related to calcium metabolism. Norman, A. W., Schaefer, K., Coburn, J. W., DeLuca, H. F., Fraser, D., Grigoleit, H. G., Herrath, D. von (eds.). pp. 637–633. Berlin: de Gruyter 1977

Henry, H. L.: Regulation of the metabolism of 25-OH-D_3: 1,25-$(OH)_2D_3$-parathyroid interactions. In: Vitamin D: biochemical, chemical and clinical aspects related to calcium metabolism. Norman, A. W., Schaefer, K., Coburn, J. W., DeLuca, H. F., Fraser, D., Grigoleit, H. G., Herrath, D. von (eds.). pp. 125–133. de Gruyter 1977

Henry, H. L., Norman, A. W.: Studies on calciferol metabolism. IX. Renal 25-hydroxy-vitamin D_3-1-hydroxylase. Involvement of cytochrome P-450 and other properties. J. Biol. Chem. *249*, 7529–7535 (1974)

Henry, H. L., Norman, A. W.: Studies on the mechanism of action of calciferol. VII. Localization of 1,25-dihydroxy-vitamin D_3 in chick parathyroid glands. Biochem. Biophys. Res. Commun. *62*, 781–788 (1975)

Henry, H. L., Norman, A. W.: Studies on calciferol metabolism. Regulation of 25-hydroxyvitamin D_3-1-hydroxylase in isolated renal mitochondria. Arch. Biochem. Biophys. *172*, 582–589 (1976)

Henry, H. L., Midgett, R. J., Norman, A. W.: Regulation of 25-hydroxyvitamin D_3-1-hydroxylase in vivo. J. Biol. Chem. *249*, 7584–7592 (1974)

Henry, H. L., Norman, A. W., Taylor, A. N., Hartenbower, D. L., Coburn, J. W.: Biological activity of 24,25-dihydroxycholecalciferol in chicks and rats. J. Nutr. *106*, 724–734 (1976)

Henry, H. L., Taylor, A. N., Norman, A. W.: Response of chick parathyroid glands to the vitamin D metabolites 1,25-dihydroxyvitamin D_3 and 24,25-dihydroxyvitamin D_3. J. Nutr. *107*, 1918–1926 (1977)

Hess, A.: The history of rickets. In: Rickets, Including Osteomalacia and Tetany. pp. 22–37. Philadelphia: Lea and Febinger 1929

Hess, A. F., Weinstock, M.: Antirachitic properties imparted to lettuce and to growing wheat by ultraviolet irradiation. Proc. Soc. Exp. Biol. Med. *22*, 5–6 (1924)

Hess, A. F., Weinstock, M., Shermàn, E.: The antirachitic value of irradiated cholesterol and phytosterol. V. Chemical and biological changes. J. Biol. Chem. *67*, 413–423 (1926)

Heymann, W.: Metabolism and mode of action of vitamin D. II. Storage of vitamin D in different tissues in vivo. J. Biol. Chem. *118*, 371–376 (1937)

Hirsch, P. F., Cooper, C. W., Peng, T-C., Burford, H. J., Toverud, S. U., Gray, T. K., Juan, D., Ontjes, D. A., Hennessy, J. F., Munson, P. L.: Effects, functions, and endocrine interrelations of thyrocalcitonin. In: Calcium Regulating Hormones. Talmage, R. V., Owen, M., Parsons, J. A. (eds.). pp. 89–99. Amsterdam: Excerpta Medica 1975

Hirschman, G. H., DeLuca, H. F., Chan, J. C. M.: Hypophosphatemic vitamin D-resistant rickets: metabolic balance studies in a child receiving 1,25-dihydroxyvitamin D_3, phosphate and ascorbic acid. Pediatrics *61*, 451–457 (1978)

Holick, M. F., DeLuca, H. F.: Chemistry and biological activity of vitamin D, its metabolites and analogs. In: Advances in Steroid Biochemistry and Pharmacology. Briggs, M. H., Christie, G. A. (eds.). pp. 111–155. London: Academic Press 1974

Holick, M. F., Schnoes, H. K., DeLuca, H. F.: Identification of 1,25-dihydroxycholecalciferol, a form of vitamin D_3 metabolically active in the intestine. Proc. Natl. Acad. Sci. USA *68*, 803–804 (1971a)

Holick, M. F., Schnoes, H. K., DeLuca, H. F., Suda, T., Cousins, R. J.: Isolation and identification of 1,25-dihydroxycholecalciferol. A metabolite of vitamin D active in intestine. Biochemistry *10*, 2799–2804 (1971b)

Holick, M. F., Garabedian, M., DeLuca, H. F.: 1,25-Dihydroxycholecalciferol: metabolite of vitamin D_3 active on bone in anephric rats. Science *176*, 1146–1147 (1972a)

Holick, M. F., Schnoes, H. K., DeLuca, H. F., Gray, R. W., Boyle, I. T., Suda, T.: Isolation and identification of 24,25-dihydroxycholecalciferol: a metabolite of vitamin D_3 made in the kidney. Biochemistry *11*, 4251–4255 (1972b)

Holick, M. F., Garabedian, M., DeLuca, H. F.: 5,6-Trans isomers of cholecalciferol and 25-hydroxycholecalciferol. Substitutes for 1,25-dihydroxycholecalciferol in anephric animals. Biochemistry *11*, 2715–2719 (1972c)

Holick, M. F., Garabedian, M., DeLuca, H. F.: 5,6-Trans-25-hydroxycholecalciferol: vitamin D analog effective on intestine of anephric rats. Science *176*, 1247–1248 (1972d)

Holick, M. F., Kleiner-Bossaller, A., Schnoes, H. K., Kasten, P. M., Boyle, I. T., DeLuca, H. F.: 1,24,25-Trihydroxyvitamin D_3: a metabolite of vitamin D_3 effective on intestine. J. Biol. Chem. *248*, 6691–6696 (1973a)

Holick, M. F., Semmler, E. J., Schnoes, H. K., DeLuca, H. F.: 1α-Hydroxy derivative of vitamin D_3: a highly potent analog of 1α,25-dihydroxyvitamin D_3. Science *180*, 190–191 (1973b)

Holick, M. F., Garabedian, M., Schnoes, H. K., DeLuca, H. F.: Relationship of 25-hydroxyvitamin D_3 side chain structure to biological activity. J. Biol. Chem. *250*, 226–230 (1975a)

Holick, M. F., Kasten-Schraufrogel, P., Tavela, T., DeLuca, H. F.: Biological activity of 1α-hydroxyvitamin D_3 in the rat. Arch. Biochem. Biophys. *166*, 63–66 (1975b)

Holick, M. F., Tavela, T. E., Holick, S. A., Schnoes, H. K., DeLuca, H. F., Gallagher, B. M.: Synthesis of 1α-hydroxy[6-^{3}H]vitamin D_3 and its metabolism of 1α,25-dihydroxy[6-^{3}H]vitamin D_3 in the rat. J. Biol. Chem. *251*, 1020–1024 (1976a)

Holick, M. F., Baxter, L. A., Schraufrogel, P. K., Tavela, T. E., DeLuca, H. F.: Metabolism and biological activity of 24,25-dihydroxyvitamin D_3 in the chick. J. Biol. Chem. *251*, 397–402 (1976b)

Holick, M. F., Frommer, J. E., McNeill, S. C., Richtand, N. M., Henley, J. W., Potts, J. T., Jr.: Photometabolism of 7-dehydrocholesterol to previtamin D_3 in skin. Biochem. Biophys. Res. Commun. *76*, 107–114 (1977)

Holst, A., Frölich, T.: Experimental studies relating ship-Beri-Beri to scurvy. II. On the etiology of scurvy. J. Hyg. *7*, 634–671 (1907)

Hopkins, F. G.: The analyst and the medical man. Analyst *31*, 385–404 (1906)

Horiuchi, N., Suda, T., Sasaki, S., Takahashi, H., Shimazawa, E., Ogata, E.: Absence of regulatory effects of 1α,25-dihydroxyvitamin D_3 on 25-hydroxyvitamin D_3 metabolism in rats constantly infused with parathyroid hormone. Biochem. Biophys. Res. Commun. *73*, 869–875 (1976)

Horsting, M.: The enzymatic conversion of cholecalciferol to 25-hydroxycholecalciferol. University of Wisconsin, Madison: Ph. D. Thesis 1970

Horsting, M., DeLuca, H. F.: In vitro production of 25-hydroxycholecalciferol. Biochem. Biophys. Res. Commun. *36*, 251–256 (1969)

Howland, J., Kramer, B.: Calcium and phosphorus in the serum in relation to rickets. Am. J. Dis. Child. *22*, 105–119 (1921)

Hughes, M. R., Brumbaugh, P. F., Haussler, M. R., Wergedal, J. E., Baylink, D. J.: Regulation of serum 1α,25-dihydroxyvitamin D_3 by calcium and phosphate in the rat. Science *190*, 578–580 (1975)

Hughes, M. R., McCain, T. A., Chang, S. Y., Haussler, M. R., Villareale, M., Wasserman, R. H.: Presence of 1,25-dihydroxyvitamin D_3-glycoside in the calcinogenic plant *Cestrum diurnum*. Nature *268*, 347–349 (1977)

Huldshinsky, K.: Heilung von Rachitis durch künstliche Höhensonne. Dtsch. Med. Wochenschr. *45*, 712–713 (1919)

Hunt, R. D., Garcia, F. G., Hegsted, D. M.: A comparison of vitamin D_2 and D_3 in New World primates. I. Production and regression of osteodystrophia fibrosa. Lab. Anim. Sci. *17*, 222–234 (1967)

Idler, D. R., Baumann, C. A.: Skin sterols. II. Isolation of Δ^7-cholestenol. J. Biol. Chem. *195*, 623–628 (1952)

Ikekawa, N., Morisaki, M., Koizumi, N., Kato, Y., Takeshita, T.: Synthesis of active forms of vitamin D. VIII. Synthesis of [24R]- and [24S]-1α,24,25-trihydroxyvitamin D_3. Chem. Pharm. Bull. *23*, 695–697 (1975)

Imawari, M., Kida, K., Goodman, D. S.: The transport of vitamin D and its 25-hydroxy metabolite in human plasma. J. Clin. Invest. *58*, 514–523 (1976)

Imrie, M. H., Neville, P. F., Snellgrove, A. W., DeLuca, H. F.: Metabolism of vitamin D_2 and vitamin D_3 in the rachitic chick. Arch. Biochem. Biophys. *120*, 525–532 (1967)

Ingersoll, R. J., Wasserman, R. H.: Vitamin D_3-induced calcium-binding protein. J. Biol. Chem. *246*, 2808–2814 (1971)

Johnson, R. L., Okamura, W. H., Norman, A. W.: Studies on the mode of action of calciferol. X. 24-Nor-25-hydroxyvitamin D_3, an analog of 25-hydroxyvitamin D_3 having "anti-vitamin" activity. Biochem. Biophys. Res. Commun. *67*, 797–802 (1975)

Jones, G., Schnoes, H. K., DeLuca, H. F.: Isolation and identification of 1,25-dihydroxyvitamin D_2. Biochemistry *14*, 1250–1256 (1975)

Jones, G., Schnoes, H. K., DeLuca, H. F.: An in vitro study of vitamin D_2 hydroxylases in the chick. J. Biol. Chem. *251*, 24–28 (1976a)

Jones, G., Baxter, L. A., DeLuca, H. F., Schnoes, H. K.: Biological activity of 1,25-dihydroxyvitamin D_2 in the chick. Biochemistry *15*, 713–716 (1976b)

Juan, D., DeLuca, H. F.: The regulation of 24,25-dihydroxyvitamin D_3 production in cultures of monkey kidney cells. Endocrinology *101*, 1184–1193 (1977)

Kanis, J. A., Heynen, G., Russell, R. G. G., Smith, R., Walton, R. J., Warner, G. T.: Biological effects of 24,25-dihydroxycholecalciferol in man. In: Vitamin D: Biochemical, Chemical and Clinical Aspects Related to Calcium Metabolism. Norman, A. W., Schaefer, K., Coburn, J. W., DeLuca, H. F., Fraser, D., Grigoleit, H. G., Herrath, D. von (eds.). pp. 793–795. Berlin: de Gruyter 1977

Kenny, A. D., Lamb, J., David, N. R., Losty, T. A.: Regulation of vitamin D metabolism in egg laying birds. Fed. Proc. *33*, 679abs (1974)

Kimberg, D. V.: Effects of vitamin D and steroid hormones on the active transport of calcium by the intestine. New Engl. J. Med. *280*, 1396–1405 (1969)

Kimberg, D. V., Schachter, D., Schenker, H.: Active transport of calcium by intestine: effects of dietary calcium. Am. J. Physiol. *200*, 1256–1262 (1961)

Kimberg, D. V., Baerg, R. D., Gershon, E., Grandusius, R. T.: Effect of cortisone treatment on the active transport of calcium by the small intestine. J. Clin. Invest. *50*, 1309–1321 (1971)

King, W. R., Francis, M. D., Michael, W. R.: Effect of disodium ethane-1-hydroxy-1, 1-diphosphonate on bone formation. Clin. Orthop. *78*, 251–270 (1971)

Kleeman, C. R., Bernstein, D., Rockney, R., Dowling, J. T., Maxwell, M. H.: Studies on the renal clearance of diffusible calcium and the role of the parathyroid glands in its regulation. In: The Parathyroids. Greep, R. O., Talmage, R. V. (eds.). pp. 353–387. Springfield: Charles C. Thomas 1961

Klein, R. G., Arnaud, S. B., Gallagher, J. C., DeLuca, H. F., Riggs, B. L.: Intestinal calcium absorption in exogenous hypercortisonism. Role of 25-hydroxyvitamin D and corticosteroid dose. J. Clin. Invest. *60*, 253–259 (1977)

Knutson, J. C., DeLuca, H. F.: 25-Hydroxyvitamin D_3-24-hydroxylase: subcellular location and properties. Biochemistry *13*, 1543–1548 (1974)

Kodicek, E.: Metabolic studies on vitamin D. In: Ciba Foundation Symposium on Bone Structure and Metabolism. Wolstenholme, G. W. E., O'Connor, C. M. (eds.). pp. 161–174, Boston: Little, Brown and Co 1956

Kodicek, E.: The metabolism of vitamin D. In: Proceedings of the Fourth International Congress of Biochemistry – Vol. 11: Vitamin Metabolism. Umbreit, W., Molitor, H. (eds.). pp. 198–208 London: Pergamon Press 1960

Kooh, S. W., Fraser, D., DeLuca, H. F., Holick, M. F., Belsey, R. E., Clark, M. B., Murray, T. M.: Treatment of hypoparathyroidism and pseudohypoparathyroidism with metabolites of vitamin D: evidence for impaired conversion of 25-hydroxyvitamin D to 1α,25-dihydroxyvitamin D. New Engl. J. Med. *293*, 840–844 (1975)

Kooh, S. W., Fraser, D., Toon, R., DeLuca, H. F.: Response of protracted neonatal hypocalcemia to 1α,25-dihydroxyvitamin D_3. Lancet *2*, 1105–1107 (1976)

Kowarski, S., Schachter, D.: Effects of vitamin D on phosphate transport and incorporation into mucosal constituents of rat intestinal mucosa. J. Biol. Chem. *244*, 211–217 (1969)

Kream, B. E., Reynolds, R. D., Knutson, J. C., Eisman, J. A., DeLuca, H. F.: Intestinal cytosol binders of 1,25-dihydroxyvitamin D_3 and 25-hydroxyvitamin D_3. Arch. Biochem. Biophys. *176*, 779–787 (1976)

Kream, B. E., Yamada, S., Schnoes, H. K., DeLuca, H. F.: Specific cytosol binding protein for 1,25-dihydroxyvitamin D_3 in rat intestine. J. Biol. Chem. *252*, 4501–4505 (1977a)

Kream, B. E., Jose, M. J. L., DeLuca, H. F.: The chick intestinal cytosol binding protein for 1,25-dihydroxyvitamin D_3: a study of analog binding. Arch. Biochem. Biophys. *179*, 462–468 (1977b)

Kumar, R., Schnoes, H. K., DeLuca, H. F.: Rat intestinal 25-hydroxyvitamin D_3- and 1α,25-dihydroxyvitamin D_3-24-hydroxylase. J. Biol. Chem. *253*, 3804–3809 (1978)

Lam, H.-Y., Schnoes, H. K., DeLuca, H. F.: 1α-Hydroxyvitamin D_2: a potent synthetic analog of vitamin D_2. Science *186*, 1038–1040 (1974a)

Lam, H.-Y., Onisko, B. L., Schnoes, H. K., DeLuca, H. F.: Synthesis and biological activity of 3-deoxy-1α-hydroxyvitamin D_3. Biochem. Biophys. Res. Commun. *59*, 845–849 (1974b)

Lam, H.-Y., Schnoes, H. K., DeLuca, H. F.: Synthesis and biological activity of 25ξ,26-dihydroxycholecalciferol. Steroids *25*, 247–256 (1975)

LaMar, G. N., Budd, D. L.: Elucidation of the solution conformation of the A ring in vitamin D using proton coupling constants and a shift reagent. J. Am. Chem. Soc. *96*, 7317–7324 (1974)

Lamm, M., Neuman, W. F.: On the role of vitamin D in calcification. Arch. Pathol. *66*, 204–209 (1958)

Larkins, R. G., MacAuley, S. J., MacIntyre, I.: Feedback control of vitamin D metabolism by nuclear action of 1,25-dihydroxyvitamin D_3 on the kidney. Nature *252*, 412–414 (1974a)

Larkins, R. G., MacAuley, S. J., Rapoport, A., Martin, T. J., Tulloch, B. R., Byfield, P. G. H., Matthews, E. W., MacIntyre, I.: Effects of nucleotides, hormones, ions and 1,25-dihydroxycholecalciferol on 1,25-dihydroxycholecalciferol production in isolated chick renal tubules. Clin. Sci. Mol. Med. *46*, 569–582 (1974b)

Larkins, R. G., MacAuley, S. J., MacIntyre, I.: Inhibitors of protein and RNA synthesis and 1,25-dihydroxycholecalciferol formation in vitro. Mol. Cell. Endocrinol. *2*, 193–202 (1975)

Lawson, D. E. M., Bell, P. A.: Metabolism of dihydrotachysterol and 5,6-trans-cholecalciferol in the chick and the rat. Biochem. J. *142*, 37–46 (1974)

Lawson, D. E. M., Wilson, P. W.: Intranuclear localization and receptor proteins for 1,25-dihydroxyvitamin D_3 in chick intestine. Biochem. J. *144*, 573–583 (1974)

Lawson, D. E. M., Wilson, P. W., Kodicek, E.: Metabolism of vitamin D. A new cholecalciferol metabolite, involving loss of hydrogen at C-1, in chick intestinal nuclei. Biochem. J. *115*, 269–277 (1969)

Lester, E., Path, M. R. C., Skinner, R. K., Wills, M. R.: Seasonal variation in serum-25-hydroxyvitamin D in the elderly in Britain. Lancet *1*, 979–980 (1977)

Liebig, J. von: Ueber die stickstoffhaltigen Nahrungsmittel des Pflanzenreichs. Ann. Chem. *39*, 129–160 (1841)

Lorenc, R., Tanaka, Y., DeLuca, H. F., Jones, G.: Calcitonin and regulation of vitamin D metabolism. Endocrinology *100*, 468–472 (1977)

MacIntyre, I., Galante, L. S., Colston, K. W., Evans, I. M. A., Larkins, R. G., MacAuley, S. J., Hillyard, C. J., Greenberg, P. B., Matthews, E. W., Byfield, P. G. H.: Regulation of vitamin D metabolism. In: Calcium Regulating Hormones. Talmage, R. V., Owen, M., Parsons, J. A. (eds.). pp. 396–404. Amsterdam: Excerpta Medica 1975

Madhok, T. C., Schnoes, H. K., DeLuca, H. F.: Mechanism of 25-hydroxyvitamin D_3 24-hydroxylation: incorporation of oxygen-18 into the 24 position of 25-hydroxyvitamin D_3. Biochemistry *16*, 2142–2145 (1977)

Magendie, F.: Ann. de Chim. et de Phys. *3*, 66 (1816). As cited in: McCollum, E. V.: A History of Nutrition. Glass, H. B. (eds.). pp. 86–87. Boston: Houghton Mifflin 1957

Maier, R.: Renal effects of human, porcine and salmon calcitonin. In: Endocrinology 1973. Taylor, S., Welbourn, R. B., Booth, C. C., Szelke, M. (eds.). pp. 184–189. London: Heinemann Medical Books 1974

Martin, D. L., DeLuca, H. F.: Calcium transport and the role of vitamin D. Arch. Biochem. Biophys. *134*, 139–148 (1969a)

Martin, D. L., DeLuca, H. F.: Influence of sodium on calcium transport by the rat small intestine. Am. J. Physiol. *216*, 1351–1359 (1969b)

Mawer, E. B.: Aspects of the control of vitamin D metabolism in man. In: Vitamin D: Biochemical, Chemical and Clinical Aspects Related to Calcium Metabolism. Norman, A. W., Schaefer, K., Coburn, J. W., DeLuca, H. F., Fraser, D., Grigoleit, H. G., Herrath, D. von (eds.). pp. 165–173. Berlin: de Gruyter 1877

McCollum, E. V., Davis, M.: The necessity of certain lipins in the diet during growth. J. Biol. Chem. *15*, 167–175 (1913)

McCollum, E. V., Simmonds, N., Pitz, W.: The relation of the unidentified dietary factors, the fat-soluble A, and water-soluble B, of the diet to the growth-promoting properties of milk. J. Biol. Chem. *27*, 33–43 (1916)

McCollum, E. V., Simmonds, N., Becker, J. E., Shipley, P. G.: Studies on experimental rickets. XXI. An experimental demonstration of the existence of a vitamin which promotes calcium deposition. J. Biol. Chem. *53*, 293–312 (1922)

Mellanby, E.: A further determination of the part played by accessory food factors in the aetiology of rickets. J. Physiol. *52*, liii (1919a)

Mellanby, E.: An experimental investigation on rickets. Lancet *1*, 407–412 (1919b)

Montecuccoli, G., Bar, A., Risenfeld, G., Hurwitz, S.: The response of 25-hydroxycholecalciferol-1-hydroxylase activity, intestinal calcium absorption and calcium binding protein to phosphate deficiency in chicks. Comp. Biochem. Physiol. *57A*, 331–334 (1977)

Moriuchi, S., DeLuca, H. F.: The effect of vitamin D metabolites on membrane proteins of chick duodenal brush borders. Arch. Biochem. Biophys. *174*, 367–372 (1976)

Moriuchi, S., Yoshizawa, S., Hosoya, N.: The effect of 1,25-dihydroxycholecalciferol on the multiple forms of alkaline phosphatase and the sialic acid incorporation into microsomes of chick duodenum. J. Nutr. Sci. Vitaminol. *23*, 497–504 (1977)

Morrissey, R. L., Wasserman, R. H.: Calcium absorption and calcium-binding protein in chicks on differing calcium and phosphorus intakes. Am. J. Physiol. *220*, 1509–1515 (1971)

Morrissey, R. L., Bucci, T. J., Empson, R. N., Jr., Lufkin, E. G.: Calcium-binding protein: its cellular localization in jejunum, kidney and pancreas. Proc. Soc. Exp. Biol. Med. *149*, 56–60 (1975)

Napoli, J. L., Reeve, L. E., Eisman, J. A., Schnoes, H. K., DeLuca, H. F.: *Solanum glaucophyllum* as a source of 1,25-dihydroxyvitamin D_3. J. Biol. Chem. *252*, 2580–2583 (1977a)

Napoli, J. L., Fivizzani, M. A., Schnoes, H. K., DeLuca, H. F.: 1α-Hydroxy-25-fluorovitamin D_3: an active analog of 1,25-dihydroxyvitamin D_3. In: Proceedings of the sixth parathyroid conference, University of British Columbia, Vancouver, Canada. Abstract 1977b, p. 64

Neer, R. M., Holick, M. F., DeLuca, H. F., Potts, J. T., Jr.: Effects of 1α-hydroxyvitamin D_3 and 1,25-dihydroxyvitamin D_3 on calcium and phosphorus metabolism in hypoparathyroidism. Metabolism *24*, 1403–1413 (1975)

Neuman, M. W., Neuman, W. F., Lane, K.: The metabolism of labelled parathyroid hormone. VI. Effects of vitamin D status. Calc. Tissue Res. *18*, 289–295 (1975)

Neville, P. F., DeLuca, H. F.: The synthesis of [1,2-^{3}H] vitamin D_3 and the tissue localization of a 0.25 μg (10 IU) dose per rat. Biochemistry *5*, 2201–2207 (1966)

Nicolaysen, R.: Studies upon the mode of action of vitamin D. II. The influence of vitamin D on the faecal output of endogenous calcium and phosphorus in the rat. Biochem. J. *31*, 106–121 (1937a)

Nicolaysen, R.: Studies upon the mode of action of vitamin D. III. The influence of vitamin D on the absorption of calcium and phosphorus in the rat. Biochem. J. *31*, 122–129 (1937b)

Nicolaysen, R.: Studies upon the mode of action of vitamin D. IV. The absorption of calcium chloride, xylose and sodium sulphate from isolated loops of the small intestine and of calcium chloride from the abdominal cavity in the rat. Biochem. J. *31*, 323–328 (1937c)

Nicolaysen, R.: Studies upon the mode of action of vitamin D. V. The absorption of phosphates from isolated loops of the small intestine in the rat. Biochem. J. *31*, 1086–1088 (1937d)

Nicolaysen, R.: The absorption of calcium as a function of body saturation with calcium. Acta Physiol. Scand. *6*, 201–209 (1943)

Nicolaysen, R., Eeg-Larsen, N.: The biochemistry and physiology of vitamin D. Vitamins Hormones *11*, 29–60 (1953)

Nicolaysen, R., Eeg-Larsen, N.: The mode of action of vitamin D. In: Ciba foundation symposium on bone structure and metabolism. Wolstenholme, G. W. E., O'Conner, C. M. (eds.). pp. 175–186. Boston: Little, Brown and Co. 1956

Nicolaysen, R., Eeg-Larsen, N., Malm, O. J.: Physiology of calcium metabolism. Physiol. Rev. *33*, 424–444 (1953)

Nordin, B. E. C.: Osteomalacia, osteoporosis and calcium deficiency. Clin. Orthop. *17*, 235–257 (1960)

Nordin, B. E. C.: The clinical significance and pathogenesis of osteoporosis. Br. Med. J. *1*, 571–576 (1971)

Nordin, B. E. C., Smith, D. A.: Diagnostic procedures and disorders of calcium metabolism. Boston: Little, Brown and Co. 1965

Norman, A. W., DeLuca, H. F.: The preparation of H^3-vitamins D_2 and D_3 and their localization in the rat. Biochemistry *2*, 1160–1168 (1963)

Norman, A. W., Midgett, R. J., Myrtle, J. F., Nowicki, H. G.: Studies on calciferol metabolism. I. Production of vitamin D metabolite 4B from 25-OH-cholecalciferol by kidney homogenates. Biochem. Biophys. Res. Commun. *42*, 1082–1087 (1971)

Norman, A. W., Friedlander, E. J., Henry, H.: Interrelationships between the key elements of the vitamin D endocrine system: 25-OH-D_3-1-hydroxylase, serum calcium and phosphorus levels, intestinal 1,25-$(OH)_2D_3$, and intestinal calcium binding protein. In: Phosphate metabolism. Massry, S. G., Ritz, E. (eds.). pp. 211–231. New York: Plenum Press 1977

O'Doherty, P. J. A., DeLuca, H. F., Eicher, E. M.: Lack of effect of vitamin D and its metabolites on intestinal phosphate transport in familial hypophosphatemia of mice. Endocrinology *101*, 1325–1330 (1977)

Offermann, G., Von Herrath, D., Schaefer, K.: Serum 25-hydroxycholecalciferol in uremia. Nephron *13*, 269–277 (1974)

Okamura, W. H., Mitra, M. N., Wing, R. M., Norman, A. W.: Chemical synthesis and biological activity of 3-deoxy-1α-hydroxyvitamin D_3 an analog of 1α,25-dihydroxyvitamin D_3, the active form of vitamin D_3. Biochem. Biophys. Res. Commun. *60*, 179–185 (1974a)

Okamura, W. H., Norman, A. W., Wing, R. M.: Vitamin D: concerning the relationship between molecular topology and biological function. Proc. Natl. Acad. Sci. USA *71*, 4194–4197 (1974b)

Okamura, W. H., Mitra, M. N., Procsal, D. A., Norman, A. W.: Studies on vitamin D and its analogs. VIII. 3-Deoxy-1α,25-dihydroxyvitamin D_3, a potent new analog of 1α,25-$(OH)_2D_3$. Biochem. Biophys. Res. Commun. *65*, 24–30 (1975)

Oldham, S. B., Fischer, J. A., Shen, L. H., Arnaud, C. D.: Isolation and properties of a calcium-binding protein from porcine parathyroid glands. Biochemistry *13*, 4790–4796 (1974)

Olson, E. B., Jr., Knutson, J. C., Bhattacharyya, M. H., DeLuca, H. F.: The effect of hepatectomy on the synthesis of 25-hydroxyvitamin D_3. J. Clin. Invest. *57*, 1213–1220 (1976)

O'Malley, B. W., McGuire, W. L.: Changes in hybridizable nuclear RNA during progesterone induction of a specific oviduct protein. Biochem. Biophys. Res. Commun. *32*, 595–598 (1968)

Omdahl, J. L., DeLuca, H. F.: Strontium induced rickets: metabolic basis. Science *174*, 949–951 (1971)

Omdahl, J. L., DeLuca, H. F.: Rachitogenic activity of dietary strontium. I. Inhibition of intestinal calcium absorption and 1,25-dihydroxycholecalciferol synthesis. J. Biol. Chem. *247*, 5520–5526 (1972)

Omdahl, J. L., DeLuca, H. F.: Mediation of calcium adaptation by 1,25-dihydroxycholecalciferol. J. Nutr. *107*, 1975–1980 (1977)

Omdahl, J. L., Gray, R. W., Boyle, I. T., Knutson, J., DeLuca, H. F.: Regulation of metabolism of 25-hydroxycholecalciferol by kidney tissue in vitro by dietary calcium. Nature (New Biol.) *237*, 63–64 (1972)

Onisko, B. L., Lam, H.-Y., Reeve, L. E., Schnoes, H. K., DeLuca, H. F.: Synthesis and bioassay of 3-deoxy-1α-hydroxyvitamin D_3, an active analog of 1α,25-dihydroxyvitamin D_3. Bioorg. Chem. *6*, 203–218 (1977a)

Onisko, B. L., Schnoes, H. K., DeLuca, H. F.: Synthesis of potential vitamin D antagonists. Tetrahedron Lett. *13*, 1107–1108 (1977b)

Orr, W. J., Holt, L. E., Jr., Wilkins, L., Boone, F. H.: The calcium and phosphorus metabolism in rickets, with special reference to ultraviolet ray therapy. Am. J. Dis. Child. *26*, 362–372 (1923)

Osborne, T. B., Mendel, L. B.: The role of the vitamines in the diet. J. Biol. Chem. *31*, 149–163 (1917)

Paaren, H. E., Hamer, D. E., Schnoes, H. K., DeLuca, H. F.: Direct C-1-hydroxylation of vitamin D compounds: convenient preparation of 1α-hydroxyvitamin D_3, 1α,25-dihydroxyvitamin D_3, and 1α-hydroxyvitamin D_2. Proc. Natl. Acad. Sci. USA *75*, 2080–2081 (1978)

Partridge, J. J., Toome, V., Uskokovic, M. R.: A stereoselective synthesis of the 24(*R*),25-dihydroxycholesterol side chain. J. Am. Chem. Soc. *98*, 3739–3741 (1976)

Partridge, J. J., Shiuey, S.-J., Baggiolini, E. G., Hennessy, B., Uskokovic, M. R.: A stereoselective synthesis of 1α,24R,25-trihydroxycholecalciferol, a metabolite of vitamin D_3. In: Vitamin D: Biochemical, chemical and clinical aspects related to calcium metabolism. Norman, A. W., Schaefer, K., Coburn, J. W., DeLuca, H. F., Fraser, D., Grigoleit, H. K., Herrath von, D. (eds.). pp. 47–55. Berlin: de Gruyter 1977

Pavlovitch, H., Garabedian, M., Balsan, S.: Calcium-mobilizing effect of large doses of 25-hydroxycholecalciferol in anephric rats. J. Clin. Invest. *52*, 2656–2660 (1973)

Pedersen, J. I., Ghazarin, J. G., Orme-Johnson, N. R., DeLuca, H. F.: Isolation of chick renal mitochondrial ferredoxin active in the 25-hydroxyvitamin D_3-1α-hydroxylase system. J. Biol. Chem. *251*, 3933–3941 (1976)

Pento, J. T., Kenny, A. D.: Mechanism of adaptation to calcium deprivation in the rat — Abstr. In: Proceedings of the 52nd meeting of the endocrine society. Endocrinol. *87* St. Louis 1970, p. 121

Peterlik, M., Wasserman, R. H.: 1,25-Dihydroxycholecalciferol-like activity in *Solanum malacoxylon*: purification and partial characterization. FEBS Lett. *56*, 16–19 (1975)

Petrova, E. A., Nikulicheva, S. I., Lazareva, N. P.: Formation of precholecalciferol in vivo. Vopr. Pitan. *5*, 50–52 (1976)

Pierides, A. M., Kerr, D. N. S., Ellis, H. A., Peart, K. M., O'Riordan, J. L. H., DeLuca, H. F.: 1α-Hydroxycholecalciferol in hemodialysis renal osteodystrophy. Adverse effects of anticonvulsant therapy. Clin. Nephrol. *5*, 189–196 (1976)

Pileggi, V. J., DeLuca, H. F., Steenbock, H.: The role of vitamin D in the prevention of rickets in rats on cereal diets. Arch. Biochem. Biophys. *58*, 194–204 (1955)

Ponchon, G., DeLuca, H. F.: The role of the liver in the metabolism of vitamin D. J. Clin. Invest. *48*, 1273–1279 (1969a)

Ponchon, G., DeLuca, H. F.: Metabolites of vitamin D_3 and their biologic activity. J. Nutr. *99*, 157–167 (1969b)

Ponchon, G., Kennan, A. L., DeLuca, H. F.: "Activation" of vitamin D by the liver. J. Clin. Invest. *48*, 2032–2037 (1969)

Popovtzer, M. M., Robinette, J. B., DeLuca, H. F., Holick, M. F.: The acute effect of 25-hydroxycholecalciferol on renal handling of phosphorus – evidence for a parathyroid hormone-dependent mechanism. J. Clin. Invest. *53*, 913–921 (1974)

Prader, A., Illig, R., Heierli, E.: Eine besondere Form der primären Vitamin D-resistenten Rachitis mit Hypocalcämie und autosomal-dominantem Erbgang: die hereditäre Pseudo-Mangelrachitis. Helv. Paediat. Acta *16*, 452–468 (1961)

Preece, M. A., McIntosh, W. B., Tomlinson, S., Ford, J. A., Dunnigan, M. C., O'Riordan, J. L. H.: Vitamin D deficiency among Asian immigrants to Britain. Lancet *1*, 907–910 (1973)

Preece, M. A., Tomlinson, S., Ribot, C. A., Pietrek, J., Korn, H. T., Davies, D. M., Ford, J. A., Dunnigan, M. G., O'Riordan, J. L. H.: Studies of vitamin D deficiency in man. Q. J. Med. New Series *19*, 575–589 (1975)

Puschett, J. B., Fernandez, P. C., Boyle, I. T., Gray, R. W., Omdahl, J. L., DeLuca, H. F.: The acute renal tubular effects of 1,25-dihydroxycholecalciferol. Proc. Soc. Exp. Biol. Med. *141*, 379–384 (1972)

Quarterman, J.: The distribution of vitamin D between the blood and the liver in the pig, and observations on the pathology of vitamin D toxicity. Br. J. Nutr. *18*, 65–77 (1964)

Raisz, L. G., Trummel, C. L., Holick, M. F., DeLuca, H. F.: 1,25-Dihydroxycholecalciferol: a potent stimulator of bone resorption in tissue culture. Science *175*, 768–769 (1972)

Rasmussen, H., DeLuca, H., Arnaud, C., Hawker, C., von Stedingk, M.: The relationship between vitamin D and parathyroid hormone. J. Clin. Invest. *42*, 1940–1946 (1963)

Rasmussen, H., Max, E. E., Goodman, D. B. P.: The effect of 1α-OH-D_3 treatment on the structure and function of chick intestine brush border membrane. In: Vitamin D: Biochemical, Chemical and Clinical Aspects Related to Calcium Metabolism. Norman, A. W., Schaefer, K., Coburn, J. W., DeLuca, H. F., Fraser, D., Grigoleit, H. G., Herrath, D. von (eds.). pp. 913–925. Berlin: de Gruyter 1977

Rasmussen, H., Pechet, M. M., Anast, C., Parks, J., Brodus, A., Bordier, P., Lane, J.: Long-term treatment of familial hypophosphatemic rickets with oral phosphate and 1α-hydroxyvitamin D_3. New Engl. J. Med. (1978) (in press)

Reed, C. I., Struck, H. C., Steck, I. E.: Vitamin D. pp. 318–319. Chicago: University Press 1939

Reeve, L. E., Schnoes, H. K., DeLuca, H. F.: Biological activity of 1α-hydroxyvitamin D_2 in the rat. Arch. Biochem. Biophys. *186*, 164–167 (1978)

Ribovich, M. L., DeLuca, H. F.: The influence of dietary calcium and phosphorus on intestinal calcium transport in rats given vitamin D metabolites. Arch. Biochem. Biophys. *170*, 529–535 (1975)

Ribovich, M. L., DeLuca, H. F.: Intestinal calcium transport: parathyroid hormone and adaptation to dietary calcium. Arch. Biochem. Biophys. *175*, 256–261 (1976)

Ribovich, M. L., DeLuca, H. F.: Effect of dietary calcium and phosphorus on intestinal calcium absorption and vitamin D metabolism. Arch. Biochem. Biophys. *188*, 145–156 (1978a)

Ribovich, M. L., DeLuca, H. F.: 1,25-Dihydroxyvitamin D_3 metabolism: the effect of dietary calcium and phosphorus. Arch. Biochem. Biophys. *188*, 164–171 (1978b)

Riggs, B. L., Gallagher, J. C.: Evidence for bihormonal deficiency state (estrogen and 1,25-dihydroxyvitamin D) in patients with post-menopausal osteoporosis. In: Vitamin D: biochemical, chemical and clinical aspects related to calcium metabolism. Norman, A. W., Schaefer, K., Coburn, J. W., DeLuca, H. F., Fraser, D., Grigoleit, H. G., Herrath, D. von (eds.). pp. 639–648. Berlin: de Gruyter 1977

Rikkers, H., DeLuca, H. F.: An in vivo study of the carrier proteins of ^{3}H-vitamins D_3 and D_4 in rat serum. Am. J. Physiol. *213*, 380–386 (1967)

Rikkers, H., Kletzien, R., DeLuca, H. F.: Vitamin D binding globulin in the rat: specificity for the vitamins D. Proc. Soc. Exp. Biol. Med. *130*, 1321–1324 (1969)

Rosenstreich, S. J., Rich, C., Volwiler, W.: Deposition in and release of vitamin D_3 from body fat: evidence for a storage site in the rat. J. Clin. Invest. *50*, 679–687 (1971)

Russell, J. E., Avioli, L. V.: 25-Hydroxycholecalciferol-enhanced bone maturation in the parathyroprivic state. J. Clin. Invest. *56*, 792–798 (1975)

Sampson, H. W., Matthews, J. L., Martin, J. H., Kunin, A. S.: An electron microscopic localization of calcium in the small intestine of normal, rachitic, and vitamin D-treated rats. Calc. Tissue Res. *5*, 305–316 (1970)

Schachter, D.: Vitamin D and the active transport of calcium by the small intestine. In: The transfer of calcium and strontium across biological membranes. Wasserman, R. H. (ed.). pp. 197–210. New York: Academic Press 1963

Schachter, D., Rosen, S. M.: Active transport of Ca^{45} by the small intestine and its dependence on vitamin D. Am. J. Physiol. *196*, 357–362 (1959)

Schachter, D., Kimberg, D. V., Schenker, H.: Active transport of calcium by intestine: action and bio-assay of vitamin D. Am. J. Physiol. *200*, 1262–1271 (1961)

Schachter, D., Finkelstein, J. D., Kowarski, S.: Metabolism of vitamin D. I. Preparation of radioactive vitamin D and its intestinal absorption in the rat. J. Clin. Invest. *43*, 787–796 (1964)

Schachter, D., Kowarski, S., Finkelstein, J. D., Wang Ma, R.: Tissue concentration differences during active transport of calcium by intestine. Am. J. Physiol. *211*, 1131–1136 (1966)

Schenck, F.: Über das kristallisierte Vitamin D_3. Naturwissenschaften *25*, 159–164 (1937)

Schneider, L. E., Omdahl, J., Schedl, H. P.: Effects of vitamin D and its metabolites on calcium transport in the diabetic rat. Endocrinology *99*, 793–799 (1976)

Schneider, L. E., Schedl, H. P., McCain, T., Haussler, M. R.: Experimental diabetes reduces circulating 1,25-dihydroxyvitamin D in the rat. Science *197*, 1 452–1 454 (1977)

Sebrell, W. H., Jr., Harris, R. S.: Vitamin D group, Chapter 7. In: The vitamins. 2nd ed. Sebrell, W. H., Jr., Harris, R. S. (eds.). pp. 155–301. New York: Academic Press 1971 Vol. 3,

Seki, M., Koizumi, N., Morisaki, M., Ikekawa, N.: Synthesis of active forms of vitamin D. VI. Synthesis of (24R)- and (24S)-24,25-dihydroxyvitamin D_3. Tetrahedron Lett. *1*, 15–18 (1975)

Semmler, E. J., Holick, M. F., Schnoes, H. K., DeLuca, H. F.: The synthesis of 1α, 25-dihydroxycholecalciferol — a metabolically active form of vitamin D_3. Tetrahedron Lett. *40*, 4147–4150 (1972)

Shah, B. G., Draper, H. H.: Depression of calcium absorption in parathyroidectomized rats. Am. J. Physiol. *211*, 963–966 (1966)

Shipley, P. G., Kramer, B., Howland, J.: Calcification of rachitic bones in vitro. Am. J. Dis. Child. *30*, 37–39 (1925)

Shipley, P. G., Kramer, B., Howland, J.: Studies upon calcification in vitro. Biochem. J. *20*, 379–387 (1926)

Sih, C. J.: Enzymatic mechanism of steroid hydroxylation. Reduced nicotinamide-adenine dinucleotide phosphate serves two distinct roles in hydroxylation. Science *163*, 1297–1300 (1969)

Silverberg, D. S., Bettcher, K. B., Dossetor, J. B., Overton, T. R., Holick, M. F., DeLuca, H. F.: Effect of 1,25-dihydroxycholecalciferol in renal osteodystrophy. Can. Med. Assoc. J. *112*, 190–195 (1975)

Spanos, E., MacIntyre, I.: Vitamin D and the pituitary. Lancet *1*, 840–841 (1977)

Spencer, R., Charman, M., Wilson, P., Lawson, E.: Vitamin D-stimulated intestinal calcium absorption may not involve calcium binding protein directly. Nature *263*, 161–163 (1976)

Stamp, T. C. B., Round, J. M.: Seasonal changes in human plasma levels of 25-hydroxyvitamin D. Nature *247*, 563–565 (1974)

Stamp, T. C. B., Round, J. M., Rowe, D. J. F., Haddad, J. G.: Plasma levels and therapeutic effect of 25-hydroxycholecalciferol in epileptic patients taking anticonvulsant drugs. Br. Med. J. *4*, 9–12 (1972)

Steele, T. H., Engle, J. E., Tanaka, Y., Lorenc, R. S., Dudgeon, K. L., DeLuca, H. F.: Phosphatemic action of 1,25-dihydroxyvitamin D_3. Am. J. Physiol. *229*, 489–495 (1975)

Steenbock, H.: The induction of growth promoting and calcifying properties in a ration by exposure to light. Science *60*, 224–225 (1924)

Steenbock, H., Black, A.: Fat-soluble vitamins. XVII. The induction of growth-promoting and calcifying properties in a ration by exposure to ultraviolet light. J. Biol. Chem. *61*, 405–422 (1924)

Steenbock, H., Black, A.: Fat-soluble vitamins. XXIII. The induction of growth-promoting and calcifying properties in fats and their unsaponifiable constituents by exposure to light. J. Biol. Chem. *64*, 263–298 (1925)

Steenbock, H., Herting, D. C.: Vitamin D and growth. J. Nutr. *57*, 449–468 (1955)

Steenbock, H. Kletzien, S. W. F., Halpin, J. G.: The reaction of the chicken to irradiated ergosterol and irradiated yeast as contrasted with the natural vitamin D in fish liver oils. J. Biol. Chem. *97*, 249–264 (1932)

Stern, P. H., Trummel, C. L., Schnoes, H. K., DeLuca, H. F.: Bone resorbing activity of vitamin D metabolites and congeners in vitro: influence of hydroxyl substituents in the A ring. Endocrinology *97*, 1552–1558 (1975)

Stern, P. H., Hamstra, A. J., DeLuca, H. F., Bell, N. H.: Bone organ culture biossay for determination of 1,25-dihydroxyvitamin D_3. In: Vitamin D.: Biochemical, chemical and clinical Aspects related to calcium metabolism. Norman, A. W., Schaefer, K., Coburn, J. W., DeLuca, H. F., Fraser, D., Grigoleit, H. G., Herrath, D. von (eds.). pp. 531–540. Berlin: de Gruyter 1977

Stohs, S. J., DeLuca, H. F.: Subcellular location of vitamin D and its metabolites in intestinal mucosa after a 10 IU dose. Biochemistry *6*, 3338–3349 (1967)

Suda, T., DeLuca, H. F., Schnoes, H., Blunt, J. W.: 25-Hydroxyergocalciferol: a biologically active metabolite of vitamin D_2. Biochem. Biophys. Res. Commun. *35*, 182–185 (1969)

Suda, T., DeLuca, H. F., Schnoes, H. K., Ponchon, G., Tanaka, Y., Holick, M. F.: 21,25-Dihydroxy-cholecalciferol. A metabolite of vitamin D_3 preferentially active on bone. Biochemistry *9*, 2917–2922 (1970a)

Suda, T., DeLuca, H. F., Schnoes, H. K., Tanaka, Y., Holick, M. F.: 25,26-Dihydroxycholecalciferol, a metabolite of vitamin D_3 with intestinal calcium transport activity. Biochemistry *9*, 4776–4780 (1970b)

Suda, T., Hallick, R. B., DeLuca, H. F., Schnoes, H. K.: 25-Hydroxydihydrotachysterol$_3$. Synthesis and biological activity. Biochemistry *9*, 1651–1657 (1970c)

Suda, T., Horiuchi, N., Fukushima, M., Nishii, Y., Ogata, E.: Regulation of the metabolism of vitamin D_3 and 25-hydroxyvitamin D_3. In: Vitamin D: biochemical, chemical and clinical aspects related to calcium metabolism. Norman, A. W., Schaefer, K., Coburn, J. W., DeLuca, H. F., Fraser, D., Grigoleit, H. G., Herrath, D. von (eds.). pp. 201–210. Berlin: de Gruyter 1977

Suda, T., Horiuchi, N., Sasaki, S., Ogata, E., Ezawa, I., Nagata, N., Kimura, S.: Direct control by calcium of 25-hydroxycholecalciferol-1-hydroxylase activity in chick kidney mitochondria. Biochem. Biophys. Res. Commun. *54*, 512–518 (1973)

Sutton, R. A. L., Harris, C. A., Wong, N. L. M., Dirks, J.: Effects of vitamin D on renal tubular calcium transport. In: Vitamin D: biochemical, chemical and clinical aspects related to calcium metabolism. Norman, A. W., Schaefer, K., Coburn, J. W., DeLuca, H. F., Fraser, D., Grigoleit, H. G., Herrath, D. von (eds). pp. 451–453. Berlin: de Gruyter 1977

Talmage, R. V.: Calcium homeostasis-calcium transport-parathyroid action. The effects of parathyroid hormone on the movement of calcium between bone and fluid. Clin. Orthop. *67*, 210–224 (1969)

Tanaka, Y., DeLuca, H. F.: Bone mineral mobilization activity of 1,25-dihydroxycholecalciferol. A metabolite of vitamin D. Arch. Biochem. Biophys. *146*, 574–578 (1971)

Tanaka, Y., DeLuca, H. F.: The control of 25-hydroxyvitamin D metabolism by inorganic phosphorus. Arch. Biochem. Biophys. *154*, 566–574 (1973)

Tanaka, Y., DeLuca, H. F.: Stimulation of 24,25-dihydroxyvitamin D_3 production by 1,25-dihydroxy-vitamin D_3. Science *183*, 1198–1200 (1974)

Tanaka, Y., Chen, T. C., DeLuca, H. F.: Dependence of 25-hydroxycholecalciferol-1-hydroxylase regulation on RNA and protein synthesis. Arch. Biochem. Biophys. *152*, 291–298 (1972)

Tanaka, Y. Frank, H., DeLuca, H. F.: Biological activity of 1,25-dihydroxyvitamin D_3 in the rat. Endocrinology *92*, 417–422 (1972a)

Tanaka, Y., Frank, H., DeLuca, H. F.: Intestinal calcium transport: stimulation by low phosphorus diets. Science *181*, 564–566 (1973b)

Tanaka, A., DeLuca, H. F., Ikekawa, N., Morisaki, M., Koizumi, N.: Determination of stereochemical configuration of the 24-hydroxyl group of 24,25-dihydroxyvitamin D_3 and its biological importance. Arch. Biochem. Biophys. *170*, 620–626 (1975a)

Tanaka, Y., Lorenc, R. S., DeLuca, H. F.: The role of 1,25-dihydroxyvitamin D_3 and parathyroid hormone in the regulation of chick renal 25-hydroxyvitamin D_3-24-hydroxylase. Arch. Biochem. Biophys. *171*, 521–526 (1975b)

Tanaka, Y., DeLuca, H. F., Akaiwa, A., Morisaki, M., Ikekawa, N.: Synthesis of 24S and 24R-hydroxy-[24-^{3}H]vitamin D_3 and their metabolism in rachitic rats. Arch. Biochem. Biophys. *177*, 615–621 (1976a)

Tanaka, Y., Castillo. L., DeLuca, H. F.: Control of the renal vitamin D hydroxylases in birds by the sex hormones. Proc. Natl. Acad. Sci. USA *73*, 2701–2705 (1976b)

Tanaka, Y., Castillo., L., DeLuca, H. F., Ikekawa, N.: The 24-hydroxylation of 1,25-dihydroxyvitamin D_3. J. Biol. Chem. *252*, 1421–1424 (1977)

Taylor, A. N.: Chick brain calcium-binding protein: comparison with intestinal vitamin D-induced calcium-binding protein. Arch. Biochem. Biophys. *161*, 100–108 (1974a)
Taylor, A. N.: In vitro phosphate transport in chick ileum: effect of cholecalciferol, calcium, sodium and metabolic inhibitors. J. Nutr. *104*, 489–494 (1974b)
Taylor, A. N., Wasserman, R. H.: Immunofluorescent localization of vitamin D-dependent calcium-binding protein. J. Histochem. Cytochem. *18*, 107–115 (1970)
Taylor, A. N., Wasserman, R. H.: Intestinal phosphate (^{32}P) absorption: effect of vitamin D and other variables. Fed. Proc. *31*, 686Abs (1972)
Taylor, S. (ed.): Calcitonin 1969. Proceedings of the Second International Symposium. London: Heinemann Medical Books 1970
Thompson, E. R., Baylink, D. J., Wergedal, J. E.: Increases in number and size of osteoclasts in response to calcium or phosphorus deficiency in the rat. Endocrinology *97*, 283–289 (1975)
Thompson, V. W., DeLuca, H. F.: Vitamin D and phospholipid metabolism. J. Biol. Chem. *239*, 984–989 (1964)
Tohira, Y., Ochi, K., Matsunaga, I., Fukushima, M., Takanashi, S., Hata, K., Kaneko, C., Suda, T.: Synthesis of 1α-[2-^{3}H]hydroxyvitamin D_3. Anal. Biochem. *77*, 495–502 (1977)
Trinh-Toan, DeLuca, H. F., Dahl, L. F.: Solid-state conformations of vitamin D_3. J. Org. Chem. *41*, 3477–3478 (1976)
Tsai, H. C., Midgett, R. J., Norman, A. W.: Studies on calciferol metabolism. VII. The effects of actinomycin D and cycloheximide on the metabolism, tissue and subcellular localization, and action of vitamin D_3. Arch. Biochem. Biophys. *157*, 339–347 (1973)
Tucker, G., III, Gagnon, R. E., Haussler, M. R.: Vitamin D_3-25-hydroxylase: tissue occurrence and apparent lack of regulation. Arch. Biochem. Biophys. *155*, 47–57 (1973)
Velluz, L., Amiard, G.: Chimie organique — le précalciférol. Compt. Rend. *228*, 692–694 (1949a)
Velluz, L., Amiard, G.: Chimie organique — equilibre de réaction entre précalciférol et calciférol. Compt. Rend. *228*, 853–855 (1949b)
Velluz, L., Amiard, G., Petit, A.: Le précalciférol: ses relations d'équilibre avec le calciférol. Bull. Soc. Chim. France *16*, 501–507 (1949)
Waddell, J.: The provitamin D of cholesterol. I. The antirachitic efficacy of irradiated cholesterol. J. Biol. Chem. *105*, 711–739 (1934)
Walling, M. W.: 1,25-Dihydroxyvitamin D_3 and intestinal phosphate absorption. In: Vitamin D: biochemical, chemical and clinical aspects related to calcium metabolism. Norman, A. W., Schaefer, K., Coburn, J. W., DeLuca, H. F., Fraser, D., Grigoleit, H. G., Herrath, D. von (eds.). pp. 321–330. Berlin: de Gruyter 1977
Walling, M. W., Kimberg, D. V.: Action of *Solanum malacoxylon* on intestine of anephric rats. Gastroenterology *69*, 200–205 (1977)
Walling, M. W., Rothman, S. S.: Phosphate-independent, carrier-mediated active transport of calcium by rat intestine. Am. J. Physiol. *217*, 1 144–1 148 (1969)
Walling, M. W., Rothman, S. S.: Adaptive uptake of calcium at the duodenal brush border. Am. J. Physiol. *225*, 618–623 (1973)
Wasserman, R. H. (ed.): The transfer of calcium and strontium across biological membranes. New York: Academic Press, 1963
Wasserman, R. H.: Calcium transport by the intestine: a model and comment on vitamin D action. Calc. Tissue Res. *2*, 301–313 (1968)
Wasserman, R. H.: Calcium absorption and calcium-binding protein synthesis: *Solanum malacoxylon* reverses strontium inhibition. Science *183*, 1092–1094 (1974)
Wasserman, R. H.: Active vitamin D-Like substances in *Solanum malacoxylon* and other calcinogenic plants. Nutr. Rev. *33*, 1–5 (1975)
Wasserman, R. H., Feher, J. J.: Vitamin D-dependent calcium-binding protein. In: Calcium binding proteins and calcium function. Wasserman, R. H., Corradino, R. A., Carafoli, E., Kretsinger, R. H., MacLennan, D. H., Siegel, S. L. (eds.). pp. 293–302. North Holland: Elsevier 1977
Wasserman, R. H., Taylor, A. N.: Vitamin D_3-induced calcium-binding protein in chick intestinal mucosa. Science *152*, 791–793 (1966)
Wasserman, R. H., Taylor, A. N.: Metabolic roles of fat-soluble vitamins D, E, and K. Ann. Rev. Biochem. *41*, 179–202 (1972)
Wasserman, R. H., Kallfelz, F. A., Comar, C. L.: Active transport of calcium by rat duodenum in vivo. Science *133*, 883–884 (1961)

Wasserman, R. H., Taylor, A. N., Fulmer, C. S.: Vitamin D induced calcium binding protein and the intestinal absorption of calcium. Biochem. Soc. Spec. Publ. *3*, 55–74 (1974)

Wasserman, R. H., Henion, J. D., Haussler, M. R., McCain, T. A.: Calcinogenic factor in *Solanum malacoxylon:* evidence that it is 1,25-dihydroxyvitamin D_3-glycoside. Science *194*, 853–855 (1976)

Weber, J. C., Pons, V., Kodicek, E.: The localization of 1,25-dihydroxycholecalciferol in bone cell nuclei of rachitic chicks. Biochem. J. *125*, 147–153 (1971)

Wells, W. W., Baumann, C. A.: Skin sterols. V. Effect of ultraviolet light on sterols of rat skin. Arch. Biochem. Biophys. *53*, 471–476 (1954)

Werder, F. von: Über Dihydro-tachysterin. Hoppe-Seyler's Z. Physiol. Chem. *260*, 119–134 (1939)

Wilson, P. W., Lawson, D. E. M.: 1,25-Dihydroxyvitamin D stimulation of specific membrane proteins in chick intestine. Biochim. Biophys. Acta *497*, 805–811 (1977)

Windaus, A., Linsert, O.: Vitamin D. Ann. Chem. *465*, 148–156 (1928)

Windaus, A., Trautman, G.: Crystalline vitamin D_4. Hoppe-Seyler's Z. Physiol. Chem. *247*, 185–188 (1937)

Windaus, A., Linsert, O., Lüttringhaus, A., Weidlich, G.: Crystalline-vitamin D_2. Ann. *492*, 226–241 (1932)

Windaus, A., Lettre, H., Schenck, F.: 7-Dehydrocholesterol. Ann. *520*, 98–106 (1935)

Wing, R. M., Okamura, W. H., Pirio, M. R., Sine, S. M, Norman, A. W.: Vitamin D in solution: conformations of vitamin D_3, 1α, 25-dihydroxy-vitamin D_3, and dihydrotachysterol$_3$. Science *186*, 939–941 (1974)

Winter, M., Morava, E., Horwath, T., Simon, G., Sos, J.: Some findings on the mechanism of adaptation of the intestine to calcium deficiency. Br. J. Nutr. *28*, 105–111 (1972)

Yamada, S., Schnoes, H. K., DeLuca, H., F.: Synthesis of 25-hydroxy-[23,24-^{3}H] vitamin D_3. Anal. Biochem. *85*, 34–41 (1978)

Zerwekh, J. E., Brumbaugh, P. F., Haussler, D. H., Cork, D. J., Haussler, M. R.: 1α-Hydroxyvitamin D_3. An analog of vitamin D which apparently acts by metabolism to 1α,25-dihydroxyvitamin D_3. Biochemistry *13*, 4097–4102 (1974)

Zerwekh, J. E., Lindell, T. J., Haussler, M. R.: Increased intestinal chromatin template activity. Influence of 1α,25-dihydroxyvitamin D_3 and hormone receptor complexes. J. Biol. Chem. *251*, 2388–2394 (1976)

Zile, M., Bunge, E. C., Barsness, L., Yamada, S., Schnoes, H. K., DeLuca, H. F.: Localization of 1,25-dihydroxyvitamin D_3 in intestinal nuclei in vivo. Arch. Biochem. Biophys. *186*, 15–24 (1978)

Zull, J. E., Repke, D. W.: The tissue localization of tritiated parathyroid hormone in thyroparathyroidectomized rats. J. Biol. Chem. *247*, 2195–2199 (1972)

Subject Index

Analogs of 1,25-dihydroxyvitamin D_3 and 25-hydroxyvitamin D_3 53–56
Assays for 1,25-dihydroxyvitamin D_3
  chromatin-binding 45
  competitive protein-binding 45
Birds
  discrimination against vitamin D_2 10
Bone
  mobilization of calcium from 49
Bone growth mechanisms
  endochondral 48
  intramembranous 48
Brush border membrane
  and calcium transport 36–37
Calcitonin 31
Calcium
  absorption of 6, 7, 35
  active transport of 35
Calcium binding protein 36–37
  effect of glucocorticoids, 37
  and vitamin D 38
Calcium homeostatic mechanism 31
Calcium metabolism
  in egg-laying birds 29
Calcium regulation of 1,25-dihydroxyvitamin D_3 production 25
Cestrum diurnum 40
Chromatin-binding assay
  for 1,25-dihydroxyvitamin D_3 45
Chylomicrons 11
Competitive protein-binding assay
  for vitamin D metabolites 45
Cytochrome P-450
  and vitamin D 25-hydroxylation 14
Cytosol receptors for 1,25-dihydroxyvitamin D_3
  in chicks 43–45
  in rats 43–45
7-Dehydrocholesterol 11–12
  chemical synthesis of 5
3-Deoxy-1,25-dihydroxyvitamin D_3 55
3-Deoxy-1α-hydroxyvitamin D_3 55
Dihydrotachysterol$_2$ 22–23
Dihydrotachysterol$_3$ 22–23
1,25-Dihydroxyvitamin D_3
  chemical synthesis of 15
  regulation of,
    by calcium 25
    by parathyroid hormone 25
1,25-Dihydroxyvitamin D_3 metabolism
  regulation by serum phosphorus concentration 28
24,25-Dihydroxyvitamin D_3 16
25,26-Dihydroxyvitamin D_3 20
Dilantin-induced osteomalacia 57
Diphosphonates
  and intestinal calcium absorption 40
  and vitamin D metabolism 40
Endogenous factor 32–33
Epiphyseal plate 48
25-fluoro-1α-Hydroxyvitamin D_3 55
Glucocorticoids
  and calcium absorption 37
  and vitamin D metabolism 40–41
25-Hydroxydihydrotachysterol$_3$ 23
24-Hydroxylation of vitamin D compounds 18–19
1α-Hydroxyvitamin D_2 54–55
1α-Hydroxyvitamin D_3 54–55
25-Hydroxyvitamin D_2 21
25-Hydroxyvitamin D_3
  chemical synthesis 15
  hydroxylation of 15
  production of 13
25-Hydroxyvitamin D_3-24-hydroxylase
  regulation of 28–29
24R-Hydroxyvitamin D_3 18
Hypocalcemic tetany in premature infants use of vitamin D compounds in treatment 58
Hypoparathyroidism
  use of vitamin D compounds in treatment 57
Hypophosphatemic X-linked dominant vitamin D resistant rickets use
  of vitamin D compounds in treatment 58
Intestinal calcium absorption
  active transport process 35–36
  response to 1,25-dihydroxyvitamin D_3 39
  response to vitamin D 35
Intestinal calcium transport 35
  mechanism of 1,25-dihydroxyvitamin D_3 action 41–43
  stimulation by phosphate transport 47
Intestinal phosphate absorption 6–7
Intestinal phosphate transport
  and vitamin D 47
Intestinal alkaline phosphatase
  and vitamin D 38

Isotachysterol vitamin D_3 23
Medullary bone resorption 30
Metabolism of vitamin D 11
Metabolites of vitamin D 17
New World monkeys
  discrimination against vitamin D_2 10
Osteomalacia 48, 58
Osteopenia 58
Osteoporosis
  glucocorticoid-induced 57
  use of vitamin D compounds therein 58
Osteosclerosis of renal failure
  use of vitamin D compounds in treatment 57–58
Parathyroid hormone
  and calcium transport 39
  and 1,25-dihydroxyvitamin D_3 25–26
  and 1-hydroxylase 19
  and 24-hydroxylase 19
  role in calcium homeostatic mechanism 33
Phenobarbital-induced osteomalacia 57
Photolysis of 7-dehydrocholesterol 11
Post-menopausal osteoporosis
  treatment with vitamin D compounds 59
  vitamin D metabolism and 59
Pseudohypoparathyroidism
  use of vitamin D compounds in treatment 57
Receptor proteins for vitamin D compounds 43–45
Regulation of vitamin D metabolism 24
Renal osteodystrophy
  use of vitamin D compounds in treatment 57
Rickets 3–4
Secondary hyperparathyroidism
  use of vitamin D compounds in prevention 57–58
Solanum glaucophyllum 40
Strontium-induced rickets 39–40
5,6-trans-Vitamin D_3 23
1,24,25-Trihydroxyvitamin D_3 18–20
Ultraviolet irradiation of skin 3
Vitamin D
  absorption of 11
  discovery of 3
  function in muscle 51–52
  as a hormone 3
  metabolism of 11
  production of in skin 11
  role in parathyroid hormone secretion 52
  storage sites 13
  and transport proteins 12
Vitamin D-dependency rickets
  use of vitamin D compounds in treatment 58
Vitamin D metabolism
  regulation of by
    estrogen 29
    progesterone 30
    testosterone 30
  and the sex hormones 29–30
Vitamin D metabolites
  biological activity of 17–18
  isolation and identification of 17–18
Vitamin D_1
  isolation of 5
Vitamin D_2 9
  discrimination against by birds 10
  discrimination against by New World monkeys 10
  isolation of 5
  metabolism of 21
Vitamin D_2 metabolites
  discrimination against by birds 22
Vitamin D_4 9

Volume 6: K. Federlin

Immunopathology of Insulin

Clinical and Experimental Studies

1971. 53 figures. XIII, 185 pages
ISBN 3-540-05408-1

Volume 5: J. Müller

Regulation of Aldosterone Biosynthesis

1971. 19 figures. VII, 137 pages
ISBN 3-540-05213-5

Volume 4: U. Westphal

Steroid-Protein Interactions

1971. 144 figures. XIII, 567 pages
ISBN 3-540-05312-3

Volume 3: F. G. Sulman

Hypothalamic Control of Lactation

In collaboration with M. Ben-David, A. Danon, S. Dikstein, Y. Givant, K. Khazen, J. Mishkinsky-Shani, I. Nir, C. P. Weller

1970. 58 figures. XII, 235 pages
ISBN 3-540-04973-8

Volume 2: K. B. Eik-Nes, E. C. Horning

Gas Phase Chromatography of Steroids

1968. 85 figures. XV, 382 pages
ISBN 3-540-04277-6

Volume 1: S. Ohno

Sex Chromosomes and Sex-Linked Genes

1967. 33 figures. X, 192 pages
ISBN 3-540-03934-1

Springer-Verlag
Berlin
Heidelberg
New York

MIX
Papier aus verantwortungsvollen Quellen
Paper from responsible sources
FSC® C105338

If you have any concerns about our products,
you can contact us on
ProductSafety@springernature.com

In case Publisher is established outside the EU,
the EU authorized representative is:
Springer Nature Customer Service Center GmbH
Europaplatz 3, 69115 Heidelberg, Germany

Printed by Libri Plureos GmbH
in Hamburg, Germany